THE MIRACLE OF BIO-IDENTICAL HORMONES

THE MIRACLE OF BIO-IDENTICAL HORMONES

"A Revolutionary Approach To Wellness
for Men, Women and Children...."

MICHAEL E. PLATT, M.D.

CLANCY LANE PUBLISHING

PLEASE BE ADVISED:

This book contains my own views and approaches to various medical conditions in men, women, and children.

It is based on years of clinical observation and feedback from my patients, and tempered by intuition and logic.

This book is not a substitute for any treatment that may have been prescribed by your physician.

Any recommendations made in this book should be discussed with your physician, who will be able to order any necessary laboratory evaluations and follow your progress, making adjustments in your treatment should they be required.

Hormones vary on an individual basis. Although natural, bio-identical hormones are safe, their misuse can produce adverse effects or consequences for which the author and publisher can not be responsible.

This book is not intended to be a medical textbook. However, it may provide you with enough information to guide you to wellness with the aid of your physician.

This book is dedicated to my mother, Bernice Platt,
whose lifelong battle with hormonal imbalance
ultimately led to her untimely death at
the age of 61 of breast cancer, and
belatedly sparked my interest
in natural hormones.

For further information, please contact:

Clancy Lane Publishing
73-345 HIGHWAY 111, Suite 203
Palm Desert, CA 92262
questions@drplatt.com
WWW.DRPLATT.COM

Book design by:

Arbor Books, Inc.
19 Spear Road, Suite 202
Ramsey, NJ 07446
www.arborbooks.com

Printed in the United States

The Miracle Of Bio-Identical Hormones:
A Revolutionary Approach To Wellness For Men, Women and Children
Michael E. Platt, M.D.

1. Title 2. Author 3. Health, Mind & Body

ISBN: 0-9776683-0-4
LCCN: 2005910810

ACKNOWLEDGEMENTS

There are many people who contributed to the making of this book. I will attempt to provide credit to them, generally in a chronological order.

My wife, Victoria, who has always been my strongest supporter and advocate, urged me to write this book. Her insight, feedback and prodding kept this book alive.

I thank my best friend, Mort Farina, a compound pharmacist, whose support I have treasured and who has made it easy for me to achieve wellness in my patients.

I received invaluable assistance from Joyce Sunila, who interviewed the patients and contributed to the format and editing of the book.

My close associate, Theresa Quintero, spent hours transcribing my scribbling into a coherent form.

Jodene Lloyd, my exceptional office manager, helped to facilitate the final birth throes of this book—expeditiously, efficiently, and noncomplainingly.

Although I do not know her, I must also give Suzanne Somers some credit for this book. The main thrust of my book was finished several years ago—and I did nothing with it until Ms. Somers' book, *The Sexy Years*, was published. After reading her book, I became aware that women had to be made aware of an alternative approach to hormone replacement besides the one she proposed. This was my strongest incentive to publish this book.

However, the most important acknowledgement I would like to give is to the thousands of my patients who have provided me with insight and feedback, allowing me to learn how to help them.

TABLE OF CONTENTS

FOREWORD

In 1962, when I graduated from Long Island University Brooklyn College of Pharmacy, botany (the study of plants) and pharmacognosy (the medicine of plants) were still being taught. Compounding pharmaceuticals was part of the mainstream curriculum. They introduced a new course, which centered on the blending of pharmacy, physiology and medicine.

With a strong background in a natural pharmaceutical approach to wellness, I was unprepared for the realities of traditional medical approaches to drug therapy.

However, in 1979 I met an amazing physician who renewed my faith in the patient-pharmacist-physician interrelationship. That physician is Michael E. Platt, M.D., a board-certified internist.

At that time in his career he was involved with a number of long term care facilities where his interest in anti-aging was ignited and where his belief in preventive medicine was reinforced. I was servicing the pharmaceutical needs of a number of the same facilities where Dr. Platt was attending. I had immediately taken note that at a time when the national average of drugs for nursing home residents averaged 9 per patient, his patients were on almost no drugs.

When we both moved to Palm Desert, California within a year of each other, we were able to re-establish the previous triad of patient—pharmacist—physician relationship. The results once again have been amazing. Dr. Platt's individual approach in treating his patients has rejuvenated my faith in the interplay of the pharmacist and physician in patient care. I was able to witness first hand the metamorphosis of his patients from sickness to wellness.

As before, he eliminates drugs where possible and continues to focus on preventive medicine. His approach to healing never ceases to amaze me as well as my fulltime staff of five pharmacists.

On behalf of my many family members whom he has unselfishly cared for and the many mutual patients we share and help,

Thank you, thank you, thank you,

Mort Farina, RPH
Compounding Pharmacist

Doctors give drugs of which they know little, into bodies of which they know less, for diseases of which they know nothing at all.

—Voltaire

CHAPTER 1

WHY THIS BOOK?

My name is Michael E. Platt, M.D. I am a board-certified internist with a practice devoted mainly to natural hormone replacement, along with wellness and metabolic weight control. I am writing this book to offer the benefit of my 33 years of clinical experience to people who are unaware of the importance of balanced hormones to health and well-being.

My fundamental approach to illness has always been from the standpoint of dealing with the cause of the illness. Since hormones control every system of the body, it is easy to see how fundamental they are to people's health. Giving a woman some Motrin for menstrual cramps may relieve the pain, but giving this woman the correct natural hormone prevents the cramps in the first place. In this book I will be dealing with a wide range of health problems that can be attributed to hormone imbalance. Some of these conditions include menopause, diabetes, asthma, obesity, migraine headaches, fibromyalgia, arthritis, cancer, fibroids, endometriosis and more.

Hormones are exceptionally powerful chemical messengers that have the ability to make you well or make you ill. They affect every cell in the body. It is fairly easy to appreciate the importance of natural hormones in terms of health maintenance, so it may be a surprise to most readers that doctors have almost no knowledge of natural hormones. Almost everything doctors learn in medical school is based on research done by pharmaceutical companies. Drug companies cannot patent natural products and thereby have no interest in spending hundreds of millions of dollars evaluating natural hormones for which they cannot receive a patent. Most endocrinologists, who specialize in hormones, do not utilize natural hormones because there are no drug companies recommending them.

I have a non-traditional approach to medicine because I deal with the cause of disease rather than the symptoms. Some people might say that I practice "alternative" medicine. However, since I utilize natural hormones, the exact hormones the body produces, I believe that I am practicing "real" medicine. Those doctors who use synthetic drugs to treat patients are, perhaps, the ones practicing alternative medicine. The term 'bio-identical' when applied to hormones simply means that the hormone is identical to the hormone produced by the body. It can be obtained by prescription from a pharmacy that is specially equipped to formulate and dispense compounded medications— i.e. a compound pharmacy. Bio-identical hormones have a natural base, most commonly soy or yam.

THE NEW (NOT SO IMPROVED) MEDICINE

The whole idea of preventing disease makes sense to most people—who can argue with it? In the old days, HMOs such as Kaiser and Ross-Loos (the first HMO in the country), were specifically formulated to provide preventive health care. In the early 1970s I worked for both organizations at various times. In those days, every lab test and procedure was covered, every medication available was on their formularies, and I was seeing only one patient per hour. Initially, HMOs were run by physicians who understood patient care. Somewhere along the way, insurance companies took over; preventive medicine was eliminated and "managed care" took its place. This perhaps was their way of saying, "what's the least amount of money we can spend and still keep the patient alive?" It's a situation that doctors and patients don't like, and pretty soon even the insurance companies won't like it as they become more and more legislated.

At this point, medicine began to change. Increasing specialization eroded the status of family practice. Insurance companies drove up prices while clamping down on the availability of lab tests. I came to feel that medicine was failing to serve the public. In particular, patients' access to appropriate preventive medicine was being sidetracked. Expensive procedures, which yield higher profits than simple remedies, became the standard of practice. Huge capital outlays were made to purchase the latest medical equipment, which then had to be justified—and sure enough, patients somehow ended up needing to utilize the equipment. Doctors became technologists. They lost interest in natural, non-invasive procedures.

Another change was that pharmaceutical companies were funding most of the major medical studies, which wound up in medical journals. Thus, the pharmaceutical companies controlled what doctors read about and also what doctors were trained to do in medical school. Their motive for underwriting these studies was not altruistic. It was part of a strategy for market dominance, similar to that of any other big business.

This book is not intended to be an exposé of American medicine. Instead, my focus is to offer a logical and sensible approach to treating various conditions, an approach that is different from traditional practices. It will provide a basic understanding of how the body operates so that one can know not only why something has gone wrong, but just as important, how to fix it.

My observations and advice in this book are based on 33 years of clinical practice. Therefore, you won't find footnotes or a bibliography or references to "double-blind" studies. None of the information here is secret, but much of it is revolutionary. Many doctors today are finding the same faults with conventional medical practice that I have found. A groundswell is starting that will, in the next 10 years, profoundly alter the way doctors go about treating patients. Most of these changes will be brought about by unhappy patients, who are a lot more educated about natural hormones than most physicians.

WHAT ABOUT MENOPAUSE?

Perhaps the one area of medicine that is the most controversial, the most mystifying, and the most inadequately approached is that of hormone replacement therapy. It is only relatively recently that women have come to question the safety of estrogen and other hormones that have been entrenched in medicine for the last 40 years.

Studies are showing that estrogen can cause aggressive cancers, heart attacks and strokes, etc. Women are being advised that they should "discuss their individual needs with their health care practitioners." However, if doctors knew anything about hormone replacement therapy, they would never have started these drugs in the first place. Often the advice these doctors give women is, "don't worry about it," or "the benefits outweigh the risks," or "it's your decision."

Into this wasteland of limited knowledge has walked a new lineup of hormone gurus who propose new alternatives. For the first time women are becoming aware of "bio-identical hormones." However, there is a tremendous misconception: that the term "bio-identical" equates with the term "safe." Nothing can be further from the truth. I will address an entire chapter on the correct use of bio-identical hormones for relief of menopausal and perimenopausal problems.

THERE'S SOMETHING WRONG

I am concerned that estrogen is still being prescribed frequently, although it is associated with six different cancers. It is recommended for patients with osteoporosis, and yet there are no studies to show that it provides a benefit to women with osteoporosis. It is recommended to help prevent heart disease and yet it is contra-indicated in coronary artery disease because the last five major studies demonstrate higher incidences of stroke and heart attack while taking estrogen. And don't forget, it is lipogenic; it creates fat and cellulite.

I am concerned that the number one drug prescribed to treat osteoporosis, other than estrogen, is also the number one source of referrals to gastroenterologists because of its toxic side effects to the gastro-intestinal tract. I am concerned that the number one drug to prevent recurrence of breast cancer, a drug that is currently being used by about 700,000 women, has never adequately demonstrated effectiveness for breast cancer prevention.

I am concerned that doctors may he blaming the wrong

hormone for prostate cancer—a condition that ultimately affects almost 100% of men if they live long enough. Throughout the book, I will address these issues and concerns. With the correct approach to hormone replacement, all of these can become non-issues.

LISTENING

One of the most common complaints I hear from patients in my office is that their doctors don't listen to them. When I did my training in medical school I was taught that 90 percent of a diagnosis is sitting down and talking to a patient. Nowadays, most doctors rush through their days trying to squeeze in as many patients as possible. They don't have time to truly listen. The average time a doctor spends with a patient is four minutes. In those instances when a doctor does listen to a patient, he winds up treating the symptoms and not the cause of the problem. So the patient is still not well.

My patients are amazed when, on their first visit, I sit down and talk to them for an hour, delving into not just their health background but the health backgrounds of their entire family. I do this for a very good reason: the more I know about my patients' bodies, their genetic history, the medications they have taken in the past, how they have responded to various interventions and so on, the better I am able to help them. By listening deeply, I can detect hormone imbalance in the particulars of people's lives; I can see clues to metabolic problems in certain kinds of behavior. My talks with patients are invaluable. Often, the lab tests I perform on my patients merely confirm what I'd already inferred from our talks.

A side benefit of our long initial conversations is that my patients develop trust. They feel attended to. Bodies are complex, intricate mechanisms. The only way to understand them is in depth. My patients sense the rightness in my habit of probing deeply into their health backgrounds. Conversely, they sense that there is something wrong when a doctor dismisses them after a four minute discussion, dispensing a one-size-fits-all treatment. They feel discounted.

The medical community has, in my opinion, become complacent. By and large, we do not show a deep personal commitment to the people who create our livelihoods. We accept all too easily that increasing numbers of our patients are overweight, that women are having miscarriages, developing breast cancer and other cancers, and that coronary artery disease and other cardiovascular ailments are running rampant. We accept the fact that many of our patients are taking multiple medications with a range of unpleasant side effects. Prescription drugs are known to be the second leading cause of death; I suspect that they may actually be the first.

Our patients are suffering, and in many cases their suffering is preventable. But before we can treat them at the cause level and ease their suffering, we must learn to listen.

HOW THIS BOOK IS ORGANIZED

Throughout this book you will meet some of my patients, telling how they felt when they came to my office and how they felt after being restored to health. As you read their case histories, you'll see how I managed to heal ailments that had been dogging my patients for years, just by balancing their hormones. Conventional doctors had treated these ailments with prescription drugs, many of which had side effects that brought on more symptoms and more disease. I was able to halt this negative progression by bringing the body's own natural endocrine system back into balance.

After my patients tell their stories, I'll comment on how I

conducted their treatment and why they got the results they received. There will be a certain amount of overlapping. Most people have multiple hormonal imbalances, so that many of my patients share similar clusters of symptoms.

Between the case histories, I've inserted brief chapters with simple, non-technical explanations on a variety of topics, including weight management. I'll talk about medications that cause weight gain and the thyroid supplements that do and don't work to regulate metabolism; i.e., information that may help readers find the key to their own weight management. Another topic puts cholesterol into perspective in order to encourage readers to become more informed. I see many practices in medicine today that aren't in patients' best interests and the only defense the public has against these practices is awareness.

There is, of course, an important chapter on bio-identical hormone treatment of the menopause in women and the andropause in men. Properly informed patients will be able to challenge their doctors and insist on proper care. One of my purposes in writing this book is to help those proactive, intelligent readers—and I know there are many of you out there, far more than there were when I first started practicing—who take pride in being conscientious, informed medical consumers.

When I consult with patients, I say things that are different from what they've heard prior to coming to me. They have often said, "Doc, you should write a book."

Well, this is that book, where I lay out what I've learned from 33 years of clinical practice. I can't prove any of the opinions I'm putting forth here, not in any way that would satisfy the demands of objective science, such as double-blind studies. But I do feel strongly about them. And I know they are sound enough to consistently create results for my patients. I include them here "for the record." Perhaps in time they'll be shown to have the scientific backing I can't claim for them today. Drs. Semmelweiss and

Lister were ridiculed in their day for suggesting that doctors wash their hands and wear gloves prior to operating on patients. They were telling doctors that they were infecting their patients, but very few believed this. Doctors, like most people, resist change.

AMAZING HORMONES

Many people are amazed to find that balancing hormones has such wide-ranging salutary (health-promoting) effects on patients. But why not? Hormones regulate every aspect of our physical being. There are thousands of receptor sites for every hormone our bodies produce, distributed over every cell of our bodies. Each receptor site has the power to alter the body's behavior in profound ways.

I believe that the benefits of natural hormone therapy should be available to everyone. That is one of the reasons for writing this book, which is designed to teach the reading public about those benefits. I am not writing this book for doctors. I am speaking to the public directly because I've seen again and again how people committed to their own health can change the system. In the past 33 years I've seen dozens of "unconventional" medical solutions brought into the mainstream by patients who insist that doctors (and insurance companies) give them what they want. I anticipate that 10 years from now, natural hormones will be standard therapy.

By writing this book, I hope to join a chorus of voices focusing attention on natural hormones. In the same way that acupuncture, herbal remedies, meditation and other "fringe" ideas have bubbled up into popular consciousness and earned credibility over the past 33 years, I would like to see natural hormone therapy come into the mainstream.

PERMANENT WEIGHT LOSS

I have placed my weight loss chapter at the end of this book for a very good reason. I don't think the world needs another diet book. I don't want this book to be confused in any way with a diet book. Saving my weight management theory for last requires that the reader develop an understanding of hormones before embarking on my weight loss program.

The reader who skips information in the early chapters of this book, intent only on finding out how to lose weight, may be disappointed. There is nothing in Chapter Twenty-Four that can help the reader lose weight until he or she understands the role of hormones in regulating metabolic health.

As you will see when you get to this chapter, I have a very different approach to weight loss. Cutting out "carbs" is not the answer to permanent weight loss. (I have observed that no matter what patients do to lose weight, sooner or later it eventually comes back on again). The reason it doesn't work is that no one deals with the underlying reasons why people gain weight in the first place. Keep in mind that hormones control every system of the body—including metabolism (weight).

My weight loss philosophy is built on the premise of discovering the underlying reason the body is creating fat. Ninety-nine percent of the time there is a hormonal problem. The majority of people with weight problems over-produce insulin. In these cases, reducing carbohydrates is mandatory. This is not a new concept—as of this writing, it is 155 years old. It is the basic approach utilized by Atkins, Sugar Busters, The South Beach Diet, The Carbohydrate Addicts Diet, Protein Power, etc. What makes my approach different is that I determine the underlying reason why the body is over-producing insulin. Failure to do so leads to the return of fat when one discontinues a low carbohydrate meal plan. This book is actually a step beyond Atkins and the South Beach Diet.

FINDING MY AUDIENCE

While writing this book I was encouraged by many people to "package" it in a way that would make it easier to sell to the general public. Some wanted me to stress my weight management work. That way the book could be marketed along with other diet books. Others felt it needed a vivid self-help formula. That would make it marketable as the next big thing for people in search of a new ray of hope in their lives.

I found it impossible to fit my ideas into these pat formulas. The book I had in me was not a diet book or a self-help book, although it does contain elements that will be useful to both groups of people. The book I had in me was what you see here—a strong point of view about the role of natural hormones in maintaining wellness, along with some maverick thoughts about the state of the healthcare industry at this time.

Despite my lack of marketing savvy, my hope is that serendipity will bring this book to the people who need it most. I will be giving exact guidelines on how to use hormones with the help of your doctor. A prescription can be obtained and filled at a compounding pharmacy. I won't publish food lists, menus, and tables (such as the glycemic index of various carbohydrates) and so on. These aids to the daily process of planning healthy meals can be found in other books. My goal here is to set forth basic principles.

"IT CAN'T BE THAT EASY"

Often after I've talked to a patient about a life-long medical problem and outlined a course of treatment, the patient responds—sometimes teary-eyed, "Doc, it can't be that easy." They've gone from doctor to doctor; they've read book after book. Many find me in the second half of their lives—their quest has gone on that long.

The tragedy is that it *is* that easy. Today's medical model has turned health care into a complex, expensive enterprise. Our specialists treat symptoms with great technical wizardry and pharmacological sophistication—while ignoring causes. Behind all the sound and fury lies a simple, overlooked truth: bodies in hormonal balance can reach a level of optimum health in a natural manner.

CHAPTER 2

BRENDA J. and ESTROGEN DOMINANCE

Brenda J., 57, visited my office primarily to discuss a weight problem. As we talked, it became clear that her "bloat," as she called it, was actually a minor factor in a constellation of symptoms whose roots were hormonal. Far more serious than her weight were complaints that had begun surfacing in her late 20's and were accelerating rapidly: an inability to focus, constant headaches, chronic fatigue, aching bones and joints, and disorientation.

I am going to let Brenda tell her story, after which I'll answer the questions you might ask if we were at a workshop together and you wanted to understand how I treated Brenda. I'll explain how unbalanced hormones hurt her and how balancing her hormones healed her. I believe her situation is not uncommon. Readers with similar afflictions may see something of themselves in the way Brenda experienced a 30-year bout with estrogen dominance.

I've had a lot of female problems since I was very, very young. My first child was born when I was 17 years old. Paul was born a severe quadriplegic with cerebral palsy. When I was 18, my second child was born and died after three months. At 22, my daughter Sandra was born. She was normal but very, very tiny: three pounds. All of my children have been born prematurely.

When I was 23 I had to have a complete hysterectomy. I had fibroid tumors and one night I went into a very severe hemorrhage and was taken to the emergency room where doctors performed the hysterectomy.

Estrogen replacement was recommended by my gynecologist after the hysterectomy. I was told I would need to take estrogen for the rest of my life, since my body no longer produced it.

As soon as I began taking Premarin I felt that something was wrong. I just didn't feel right. I told my gynecologist about this feeling and I suggested it might be the estrogen. But he told me that wasn't the problem, and that I had to be on estrogen. That was when I began gaining weight.

For the first five years after my hysterectomy my only symptom was this gradual weight gain. But then other symptoms began appearing. I began feeling fuzzy in the head. My vision started to blur, I wasn't sleeping well and my joints started hurting.

When my first gynecologist retired another doctor took over his practice. I tried talking to this doctor too, telling him how I felt. But he had the same reaction to my complaints as the first doctor. In fact he thought my symptoms indicated that I might not be getting enough estrogen and he increased my dosage. This doctor put me on Synthroid, a thyroid drug, and kept increasing the amount of Premarin I was

*taking, so that by the time I was in my 40's I'd been taking 2.5mg,
the maximum dosage of Premarin, for about 10 or 12 years. The gynecologist would explain away my depression by saying, "Of course you're
depressed. You have a handicapped child. You had a child that died.
Your depression is normal."*

*I got divorced in my 30s and about a year after the divorce my
physical problems started in earnest: the aches and pains, the fuzzy
thinking, the deep fatigue, headaches, and of course the bloated body
which got worse every year. I honestly don't know how I managed back
in those days after the divorce. I was so exhausted all the time I didn't
know which end was up.*

*A typical day would start with me getting up and my body hurt-
ing so badly that I would get into the shower and stand under the hot
water until I could bend my arms and legs and move a little. Then I
would get dressed and I was already exhausted. But somehow I'd do
my work; you just do what you have to do.*

*During this whole time I tried getting second, third and fourth
opinions about the Premarin from various gynecologists. When I moved
to Lake Arrowhead, California, I tried a gynecologist there. This doctor told me to keep taking the Premarin and that the only problem I
had with weight was that I had to stop eating so much. I told him "I
don't eat. I starve myself to death and I exercise until I fall on my face
and almost pass out." He said, "Well, I never saw a fat woman in a
concentration camp." I got so mad I got up and walked out of his office.
Shortly after that I read about this program at Duke University where
you could get a total medical work-up. I flew to Raleigh, N. C. and
entered the program. I filled out endless forms and had blood tests and
a hormone panel and all kinds of testing done. I lived there for six
weeks and spent almost $20,000.*

*At the end of the whole thing they told me there was nothing
wrong with me and that I should go home and visit a psychiatrist. It
was the same old song: you've had a hard life; you're stressed out; keep
taking your Premarin and see a counselor.*

The doctors at Duke University increased my dosage of Synthroid and put me on a high-carbohydrate diet. I was eating bagels and fruit in the morning, pasta for lunch and dinner, and now I started really bloating out. My metabolism was slowing down even more. I have photographs of myself from this period and it takes my breath away to look at them. I was so huge! I was a size 14.

I developed a new symptom. I started having disoriented moments where I'd be on the freeway and I couldn't remember where I was going or why I was there.

The turnaround came when I talked to a woman who was having some of the same problems I was having—achy joints, weight gain, puffiness, fatigue. We'd commiserate with each other, blaming it on our age. "Getting old isn't what it's cracked up to be," we'd tell each other. Then I didn't see her for about four or five months and one day I was out walking my dog and ran into her. I hardly recognized her. "My God, what are you doing?" I asked her. She told me about Dr. Platt, and I went to see him the following week.

The first thing I noticed about Dr. Platt was that he really listened to me. Most doctors don't hear you, but Dr. Platt makes you feel like you're talking to your best friend. He did my hormone panel and told me he was taking me off Premarin. My first reaction was shock. All of my life doctors had been telling me that I needed estrogen replacement. I thought, "Maybe this isn't going to work." A few times I'd tried to wean myself from Premarin and the hot flashes and headaches were unbearable.

And the way he was telling me to eat! Meats and vegetables, bacon and eggs for breakfast—it went against everything the culture was telling us about cholesterol and everything else. But at the end of our first meeting he said something that made me trust him. He said, "None of this is your fault. You've just never received proper treatment."

So I started taking progesterone, two different thyroid hormones and eating what he told me to eat. I was eating meat, eating eggs, eating three meals a day. I never ate so much in my life. And the results happened so fast I couldn't believe it. I could just see daily where the weight dropped. And my energy shot up. I don't ever remember feeling the way I started to feel. I felt wonderful and happy and energetic.

I can't even describe it, it all happened so fast. I was thinking clearly, my vision cleared up, my headaches stopped, I started sleeping at night. In about a month I had to buy a new wardrobe. I immediately got rid of everything in size 14. I went down to a size four in two months.

The aches and pains started going away gradually. At six months I realized that my arms didn't hurt. I could get up in the morning and move my arms.

By this time I felt so great that my husband couldn't keep up with me. I had more energy than he could handle. So he went to see Dr. Platt and he got amazing results, too. He's 11 years older than me and has always been very healthy, but now he feels like 40 again.

When I see friends they're shocked at how well I look. They think I've lost 90 pounds (I've actually only lost 47 pounds). My vitality is unlike anything they've seen in me before.

You know, when it comes right down to it, it isn't even the difference in how you look...it is how you feel. I wouldn't give up how I feel for anything.

MIRACLE OR SIMPLE CHEMISTRY

The transformation Brenda J. testifies to may sound incredible, but the truth is that it's not an unusual occurrence in my practice. I attribute every bit of it to the power of hormones. They regulate activity in every cell in the body, including brain cells. As miraculous as Brenda's healing sounds, it was no miracle— it was a matter of chemistry, pure and simple.

In the beginning, Brenda came to me showing all of the classic signs of estrogen dominance. She'd been laboring under the weight of excess estrogen her entire life, even before she was prescribed estrogen in the form of Premarin in her 20's. The reason for her overproduction of estrogen was a lack of progesterone. This deficiency of progesterone was the major cause of her problem pregnancies, and certainly the cause of her fibroids, which ultimately resulted in the need for a hysterectomy.

Just putting her on bio-identical natural progesterone made her feel better right away. Progesterone is a natural anti-depressant; it's the feel-good hormone for women. With the proper amount of progesterone in her body, Brenda's mood brightened. Progesterone is the hormone that balances out estrogen and takes away its worst side effects.

Progesterone is also thermogenic. It helps fat to burn by helping the thyroid gland to function better, as well as by raising body temperature. And it helps prevent the overproduction of insulin, the main hormone that creates fat and keeps it stored. So Brenda's metabolism improved and she began to see her weight melting away.

She was more comfortable inside her own body. That alone had to make her feel much, much better. Her fatigue started lifting, too. She had energy she didn't have before.

Part of her weight loss was related to a reduction in fluid retention which had been created by too much estrogen, too much insulin and the wrong thyroid medication.

STANDING UP TO ESTROGEN DOMINANCE

The improvement I saw in Brenda just a month or two after starting her on progesterone is something I see again and again in my practice. What people have to understand is that in many cases estrogen is toxic to the body. You can think of progesterone as an anti-estrogen hormone. Progesterone is there to protect the body from the negative effects of estrogen.

Which negative effects? Estrogen is very damaging to blood

vessels. This is why it causes migraine headaches. Doctors are very much aware of estrogen's effect on blood vessels. It's why they warn women on birth control pills to be on the lookout for any signs of phlebitis, which is an inflammation of the veins. Birth control pills contain two synthetic hormones—an estrogen and a progestin.

Estrogen causes six different cancers in women. It's been known for over 50 years that estrogen causes breast cancer. Except for the drug Tamoxifen, to my knowledge estrogen is the only known cause of cancer of the uterus and probably the only known cause of cancer of the ovaries. It is also a cause of cervical cancer, vaginal cancer and cancer of the colon.

Every two years an effort was made to place estrogen on the list of cancer-causing chemicals. Once a drug is on this list special warnings are supposed to be given. Estrogen finally got on this list in 2003; however, you wouldn't know it.

I am not the first doctor to point out the overuse of estrogen in medicine today. The term "estrogen dominance" was coined by Dr. John R. Lee in his 1996 book, *What Your Doctor May Not Tell You About Menopause*. He was the first M.D. to go public decrying the use of estrogen to "cure" women's menopause.

Unfortunately, the concept of estrogen dominance is not widely accepted in the medical community. In fact, many doctors have very little understanding of hormones at all. This is a topic I'll come back to again and again. It's one of the primary themes of this book—the conventional medical community is largely unaware of how important hormones are in regulating every aspect of our physical well being, or rather they understand it intellectually, but do not apply it to their practices.

Doctors were never taught in medical school that there's such a thing as too much estrogen. To the medical community there's no such thing as a disease caused by too much estrogen. They know that there are conditions called fibroids and endometriosis, they know that women get fibrocystic disease in their breasts and so on, but they don't seem to be concerned about estrogen's role in causing these conditions. Women with these problems should never be given estrogen because they are at risk for even more serious complications of estrogen dominance.

Morning sickness is only caused by too much estrogen. But doctors don't realize that. They don't know that you can prevent morning sickness and that you can prevent miscarriages by prescribing bio-identical progesterone. Natural hormones can help women with common problems like these, but doctors are generally unaware of it.

It is very difficult for people, doctors included, to separate the hype associated with estrogen from the reality. Most of the research on estrogen has been bought and paid for by drug companies who have almost 100 percent control over what gets published and, more importantly, what doesn't.

It's been proposed by drug companies, and by the doctors who tend to believe what these companies have to say, that estrogen is good for the heart. And yet five major studies have indicated that women starting on estrogen have higher incidences of heart attacks and strokes. Estrogen is now contraindicated in women with coronary artery disease and women who have had strokes. The American Heart Association is now telling doctors to be much more selective in giving women estrogen.

In this regard, a negative side effect of estrogen is that it elevates homocysteine levels, the substance that makes blood vessels sticky, leading to clot and plaque formation.

Estrogen is always promoted for the treatment of osteoporosis, and it appears that in some studies it may give a temporary benefit for the prevention of osteoporosis. There have been no studies to show that estrogen reverses osteoporosis. It is primarily a lack of progesterone that causes osteoporosis.

Studies are now finding that women on birth control pills, which suppress progesterone production, have earlier onset of osteoporosis.

In women, progesterone is one of the hormones of choice in the treatment of osteoporosis. It stimulates osteoblasts in the bone to make new bone. Estrogen does not do this.

THE HEALING POWERS OF PROGESTERONE

When you realize that there are over 300 receptor sites for progesterone throughout the body, it gives you an idea of the powerful effects patients can experience when they are given progesterone.

In general, progesterone is wonderful for brain tissue. In fact, progesterone levels are higher in brain tissue than anywhere else in the body. So it influences memory function, and there have been studies to indicate it's very good for preventing and possibly even treating Alzheimer's disease.

It's also wonderful for nerve tissue. I've used it with diabetics who have a burning neuropathy in their feet. Sometimes within three days the neuropathy is gone. It stimulates Schwann cells that line the axis of nerves to produce myelin. Multiple sclerosis is a condition associated with the demyelinization of nerve cells. Most of the patients I have seen with MS have been estrogen dominant. Could this condition possibly be related to low progesterone levels?

It also has a healing effect on blood vessels. It undoes all the damage that estrogen does. That's why it works so well for preventing and treating menstrual migraines, and why it's effective in preventing coronary artery spasm.

It's one of the best treatments for osteoporosis. It's much better than estrogen in that regard. And because progesterone reduces insulin levels—the number one hormone that creates fat in most people—it can be used to help control weight.

Progesterone is also a natural anti-depressant. It's a feel-good hormone, especially for women. As the antidote to estrogen, it helps prevent breast cancer, cancer of the ovaries and probably cancer of the colon. It prevents cancer of the prostate because, I also feel, that is another cancer caused by estrogen.

Brenda would have had a completely different life if the benefits of progesterone were understood by the medical community. Instead, she was estrogen dominant, which led to her hysterectomy and brought on a surgically induced menopause. At that point, Brenda became a victim of the Premarin trend, also known as Estrogen Replacement Therapy. It began in earnest in the 1970s. Before the 1970s, there was nothing in the gynecological canon that dictated giving women estrogen at menopause. I will be discussing the roots of hormone replacement therapy in the chapter on the menopause.

FIBROMYALGIA

The pain in her joints that Brenda began to experience in her 30s was not caused by estrogen. In my practice I come across many patients in whom physical pain—arthritis, fibromyalgia and so forth—is intermixed with their symptoms of hormone imbalance. Just getting hormones in balance often leads to relief of fibromyalgia.

For the most part these people are angry. Their hormone imbalances are allowed to go on year after year. They take part in expensive, time-consuming efforts to treat their symptoms, and the symptoms stubbornly persist. It's understandable that they'd develop anger about their lot in life.

Anger can cause muscles to tense. When you tense a muscle

it produces lactic acid that causes pain, and the persistent tensing of the muscles utilizes a lot of energy, which causes fatigue. The way I treat patients with fibromyalgia is to deal with the underlying cause of their anger and to get hormones back in balance.

I will be addressing fibromyalgia in Chapter 16. I've found this condition to be present in many of the people who seek out my services and, as with Brenda, it is usually not properly diagnosed.

Although Brenda doesn't mention it, she was operated on for TMJ, or pain in the temporal mandibular joint. She told me this in our intake interview. TMJ is caused by tensing of the jaw muscles, which occurs usually at night, and is always associated with anger.

Brenda had a lot of good reasons to be angry. She was being misled by the medical community and she had—let's face it— a hard life raising her children on her own. I find her situation almost tragic. Here she was crying out for help, exhibiting classic symptoms that should have been impossible to miss, yet no one would listen to her.

I can't emphasize enough the importance of utilizing hormones correctly. Some women are more sensitive to foreign substances than others. Brenda was a woman who sensed something wrong the moment Premarin was introduced into her system. She communicated this to her doctor but he refused to give credence to her intuition. Ironically, when she tried to wean herself off Premarin she suffered hot flashes and headaches. This is because foreign substances, once they are established on the cellular level, are difficult to flush out. For many women, coming off Premarin is like coming off heroin. A woman can go through severe withdrawal headaches, nausea, hot flashes, night sweats, etc.

It is felt that hot flashes may be caused by luteinizing hormone, a hormone that is secreted by the pituitary gland. The pituitary sends this hormone to stimulate the ovaries to produce estrogen or progesterone or other hormones. It's luteinizing hormone that produces the vasomotor effects that women get; i.e., hot flashes and night sweats. Anything that elevates luteinizing hormone will produce hot flashes.

This can be caused by a lack of estrogen, progesterone, and perhaps even testosterone. Taking someone off estrogen leads to an increase in luteinizing hormone, which can precipitate hot flashes.

Sometimes the pituitary is reacting to the fact that progesterone is low. So just giving progesterone can take away hot flashes.

Balancing people's hormones is a very delicate juggling act. You have to fine-tune hormones. Working with a compounding pharmacist makes it easier.

In another chapter I will address the weaning from Premarin.

WHY DUKE UNIVERSITY FAILED

The medical center at Duke University is one of the most respected medical centers in the world. Brenda went there and told them that she just didn't feel good, so they put her through $20,000 worth of testing and at the end of six weeks said, basically, "There's nothing wrong with you. You have to speak to a psychiatrist."

How could this happen? How could they have failed to diagnose her properly after *$20,000 worth of tests?*

One factor in their failure is something I witness over and over again among conventional doctors: they don't treat patients, they treat lab tests. Nobody sits down and talks to patients any more. If they did, it would have been hard for them to miss the constellation of symptoms Brenda was exhibiting.

When most doctors do blood tests they don't always test for hormones. If they do, they don't always test for the correct hormones. I didn't need to do any blood tests on Brenda to know that she had hormone problems. In fact, I would have treated her without doing blood tests, her symptoms were so classic.

It's not surprising to me that a center like Duke could miss Brenda's symptomatology. Unfortunately, they're part of the medical establishment. Medicine is for the most part very traditional and when you talk about natural hormone replacement, you're out on the fringes.

The doctors at Duke University are not bad doctors. Most of them are academically inclined and simply won't believe nontraditional approaches that have not been verified by double-blind studies. Universities, and the hospitals and clinics associated with them, tend toward medical conservatism. They're also heavily influenced by pharmaceutical companies. The pharmaceutical companies fund all the big medical studies, creating an aura of legitimacy around their products. In these settings, doctors' view of the wellness movement and natural products is skewed. They tend to dismiss both.

AN UNDERACTIVE THYROID

Excess estrogen and low progesterone weren't Brenda's only hormone problems. She also had an underactive thyroid. Once her body received the correct type and dose of thyroid supplement, her metabolism increased and she was able to burn fat. She had more energy. As her fat reserves shrank, she felt lighter and more optimistic.

The doctors at Duke University diagnosed Brenda with an

underactive thyroid, but they utilized the wrong thyroid approach. Doctors, for the most part, fail to realize there are two different thyroid hormones and both have to be assessed. In spite of $20,000 worth of testing, they failed to realize that she was not making enough liothyronine (T3)—the thyroid hormone responsible for 90% of the activity of the thyroid. They gave her Synthroid, which is thyroxine (T4), basically a storage hormone. T4 must be converted to T3 to be effective, but Brenda's body was unable to convert T4 into T3, so Synthroid was ineffective for her. This is something I'll go into in more detail in Chapter Three.

We're also to some extent looking at the influence of the pharmaceutical companies here. Synthroid is so well-publicized that it's all that most doctors know when it comes to supplementing the thyroid gland.

Six weeks after she first came to my office, Brenda came in and we sat down and talked. "Doc," she said, "I've never felt better in my entire life." That shows you the power of hormones.

AN OUNCE OF PREVENTION

To my mind, Brenda's life and her battle with estrogen teach one very important lesson: it's easier to prevent disease than it is to cure it. That's why it's essential that doctors educate themselves about hormones. They're foundational. If you can balance a patient's hormones, you can often treat their problems at the source without resorting to surgery and drugs. Brenda is a perfect example of the miraculous power of bio-identical hormones.

CHAPTER 3

THE TWO TYPES of THYROID HORMONES

The thyroid gland controls metabolism in every cell of the body. A thyroid deficiency can cause a multitude of symptoms in the body, the classic ones being weight gain, dry skin, poor nails, low body temperatures, sluggishness and memory problems. Thyroid hormone controls the rate at which calories are burned to produce energy. Dr. Atkins has stated that the number one reason for "metabolic resistance"—the term he uses to describe the inability to burn fat—is a thyroid deficiency.

THE WRONG THYROID HORMONE

Although most people don't realize it, there are actually two thyroid hormones, T3 and T4. The thyroid gland produces and releases T4, which goes to the liver where it is converted into T3. By itself, T4 does not do most of the tasks of the thyroid hormone—it is essentially a storage hormone. T3 is the active form of thyroid, and it is responsible for most, but not all, of its functions. Obviously, any problem resulting in a lack of T3 will create low thyroid symptoms.

Unfortunately, in the medical community today the primary attention in terms of testing and treating thyroid disorders is paid to T4. Doctors test for T4 and regard it as the barometer of a person's metabolic health. What they don't realize is that a person can have a perfectly normal T4 level and still be hypothyroid (lacking in sufficient thyroid hormone) because of an inability to convert T4 to T3. Unless a patient can convert T4 into T3, their bodies will lack the essential ingredient for a properly acting metabolism.

The most commonly prescribed medications for low thyroid conditions are Synthroid and Levoxyl. Both are T4 preparations. This means that most people who exhibit low thyroid symptoms are prescribed something that may or may not address their problem. In my practice I constantly come across patients who have been taking Synthroid for years without getting any relief from their symptoms of a low-functioning thyroid. Their doctors continue to prescribe the T4 preparation regardless of its lack of results because of normal T4 levels on blood tests. As I've said before, many doctors treat blood tests instead of patients.

There are T3 preparations available which, for the most part, are ignored by the medical community.

Aggravating the problems is a number of medications that interfere with thyroid metabolism, preventing or slowing the conversion of T4 into T3. These include cholesterol-lowering statin type drugs such as Lipitor and Zocor, which lower coenzyme Q10, a factor necessary for thyroid conversion. I will talk about these again in my chapter on the medications that prevent weight loss.

Ironically, one of the most common reasons for an elevated cholesterol level is an under active thyroid. This means that many people are being prescribed a thyroid-blocking drug for the purpose of treating a condition that may be caused by an underactive thyroid in the first place. When I see people with high cholesterol, my first thought is that they might be low in thyroid. In the old days, they used to call cholesterol "the poor man's thyroid test."

Beta-blockers such as Atenolol, Ziac, Lopressor, etc., also block the conversion of T4 into T3. These drugs are commonly used by cardiologists for their heart patients to reduce the workload of the heart. However, they almost guarantee weight gain, which is—ironically—one of the most significant risk factors for coronary artery disease.

THYROID STIMULATING HORMONE

I apologize if it seems as though we're getting a little technical, but it is my feeling that there are millions of people who are improperly treated, or not treated at all, for an underactive thyroid condition. I think the reasons for this are twofold: the failure of many doctors to listen to what their patients are saying and the failure to interpret laboratory tests logically.

TSH, also known as Thyroid Stimulating Hormone, is considered the most sensitive of all thyroid tests by most doctors—in fact, it's often the only thyroid test that's ordered. If the pituitary gland detects suboptimal thyroid levels it sends out TSH to stimulate the thyroid to make more hormones. They have established "normal" levels as falling between the ranges of 0.3 to 5.5. If your TSH level is within this range, your test is considered normal and no thyroid will be prescribed. However, the fact is that any TSH level greater than 1.0 can be your pituitary saying "you need thyroid." The normal range was arbitrarily established by determining the TSH levels of a 100 medical students with no concern as to how their thyroids functioned.

Doctors always wait for the TSH level to go higher than 5.5. By that time, patients are severely hypothyroid. My goal when I treat patients is to get the TSH level close to 0.3—at this point I know they are getting close to 100% of the thyroid they require. However, I use two different thyroid hormones to achieve this—both T3 and T4. A low TSH using only Synthroid or Levoxyl may indicate the possibility of too much medication, and is often associated with a higher than normal heart rate.

WHAT YOU CAN DO

A proper thyroid evaluation should include a history evaluation and the proper tests. Signs and symptoms of low thyroid include: dry skin (without using moisturizers), brittle or soft nails, cold feet, blood clots with periods, low body temperature, fatigue, poor memory, dry, brittle hair and elevated cholesterol.

Sensible thyroid testing would include:

Free T4

Free T3

TSH

Note: Free T4 and Free T3 do not mean there is no charge. These tests measure unbound thyroid that is biologically active and not affected by levels of thyroid binding globulin.

T3 PREPARATIONS

To my way of thinking, proper thyroid dosing might include both thyroid hormones.

There are various T3 preparations, including Armour, Thyrolar and Cytomel. The first two include combinations of T3 and T4. However, the T3 is short-acting (three hours) and they never have enough T4. Cytomel is synthetic T3 and is also short-acting.

My preference is giving a sustained-release form of natural T3 once or twice a day. This can be obtained through a compound pharmacy. To this I would add the proper dose of L-thyroxin (Levoxyl or Synthroid).

For those of you that are interested, there will be a special chapter on how and when to do hormone testing and how to determine proper dosages based on symptoms and results of your lab tests.

CHAPTER 4

RHONDA Y. and HORMONAL FATIGUE

Fatigue is a common symptom in bodies that have gone out of balance. For Rhonda Y., 38, hormonally induced fatigue had eroded the joy of raising her family. Fortunately, I was able to help her regain hormonal balance, restoring her zest for living and a full life with her loved ones. But how many chronically fatigued homemakers stumble through the daily grind of the caregiver's life, branded as hypochondriacs and failing to receive help?

I've chosen to include Rhonda in this book because I find something frightening in the way the medical system failed her and fails people like her every day.

My medical problems began early, with pains in my pelvic area that would get so bad I would be doubled over. My first pregnancy was an ectopic pregnancy. That's a pregnancy in which the fetus develops in the fallopian tubes and I had to have surgery for that. Later I had endometriosis, and went through several operations for that. My two sons were conceived through the expensive and painful method of in vitro fertilization.

At age 31 my whole system started taking a dive. That was when the weight gain started. I had always been a normal weight but suddenly I started putting on pounds. Along with the weight came a host of new symptoms.

One was asthma. Another was acid reflux, which was very painful, and then a third painful condition, irritable bowel syndrome. I developed high blood pressure and also had a kidney infection. These were all debilitating conditions, but the worst of it was a new level of fatigue that hit me, that made raising my children a kind of daily torment.

The fatigue went on all day but it would hit me hard at about 7 or 8 o'clock at night, at which time I just couldn't do anything. I pretty much set my bedtime at 8 p.m. The fatigue made domestic chores impossible to complete. I needed to rest a lot during the day. The messes around the house began to seem like mountains I had to climb. The kids' demands were constant and I lost my cheerfulness early in the day. I yelled a lot and felt constantly irritable.

Often I couldn't face putting a big meal on the table in the evening and cleaning up afterwards, so I'd take the kids out for fast food. (My husband didn't come home until 8 or 9 o'clock at night). I was craving caffeine and sugar to give myself a lift, and I could get those at a fast food place. I felt guilty about not giving my kids whole foods, but by the time evening came around I often felt too tired to care. Luckily, I'm blessed with wonderful kids that were aware of my problem and learned how to take care of themselves.

I was just getting by as a mother, doing the bare minimum. The area where there was the most fallout was in recreation and social activities. Once I'd taken care of the necessities, I just didn't have the energy for anything more. My husband would take the kids places on Sundays but I never went with them; I was so relieved just to be able to rest and not have anyone asking me for anything. The kids got used to playing with their dad and not expecting mom to be there.

As far as socializing with other families went, I didn't have what it took to prepare meals and entertain. We were isolated. My husband compensated by socializing with his family, who live close by. I enjoy my husband's family but I rarely went with him and the kids. I just wanted to rest.

I went to a lot of doctors about the fatigue. They all said there was nothing they could do about it. Most of them were condescending and treated me like a child or some kind of mental case.

My husband was constantly concerned about my health and what was going on with me. Our sex life had come to a standstill. I had no sex drive. It could have been because of the 20 milligrams of Paxil that I was taking for my depression. Or it might have been the blood pressure medication, which I took in high doses. Or it could have been plain old fatigue. You don't feel much like having sex when all you want to do is lie down and rest.

What with all of my ailments and the depression and the fatigue, I started to think my life was coming to an end. Family life had become nothing but domestic tasks, and it seemed as though every week my body was failing in another way. I was on medication for depression but it didn't help because I had this sense of impending doom. I wondered what would happen next that would cause me to be put on even more medication. I was unsure and frightened.

One day I was talking with the therapist I saw for my depression and she mentioned that she had some other clients who'd benefited from going to The Compounding Pharmacy in Palm Desert and getting natural hormone therapy. I went there and they recommended I see Dr. Platt. Since I had been to at least 25 or 30 doctors, I was a little skeptical about seeing Dr. Platt. But my desperation gave me no choice.

Soon after I went in for my intake interview I started the meal plan and I got off caffeine and sugar. A week later I started taking DHEA, progesterone, testosterone and a T3 thyroid preparation. Dr. Platt told me about the Synthroid I'd been taking for years, which previous doctors had prescribed for my low thyroid. He explained to me that my body was unable to convert Synthroid's T-4 into T-3, which is the actual thyroid hormone that does all the metabolic work of the thyroid gland. Apparently I'd been taking Synthroid all those years and it hadn't been doing anything for me.

My energy level increased drastically. Between the hormones, the increase in protein, the diet in general and the removal of medications that had been throwing my body off balance, I found a big difference in my ability to function.

Once I had more energy I wasn't as grouchy or impatient as I used to be. I was able to deal with things better both emotionally and physically. The best part has been my ability to participate with my family more.

Whereas I used to let my husband take the children out while I stayed home and rested, now I can participate in family outings. Our church has volleyball twice a month and now I enjoy playing that with my family. We go walking and sightseeing. My children are so happy that mom can go places with them now; I think they feel comfortable that mommy will be there with them.

Also, before we had no social life as a family. Now we try to have guests visit the house twice a month to eat with us. My husband and I go out with other couples more often. I also see his family more, which I enjoy.

Being able to socialize again, especially with my family, has been so wonderful. For something so simple, it's astonishing.

THE ROOTS OF FATIGUE

Let's talk about fatigue. It came very close to ruining Rhonda's home life. She went to doctor after doctor and no one could help her. Does that sound familiar? If it does, you're not alone. In my practice I meet many women who go to bed exhausted and wake up tired. They've lost their zest for life and they feel inadequate to the demands of a normal life.

Rhonda's fatigue was caused by multiple factors. All of them were influenced by an imbalance of hormones. The main source of her fatigue was fibromyalgia—again, a very common condition and mostly ignored by the medical community. The number one hormone associated with this condition is thyroid. Just getting thyroid into balance often leads to a reduction in symptoms.

Another cause of her fatigue was recurrent hypoglycemia. A condition caused by the overproduction of insulin often caused by a lack of progesterone. Anytime insulin levels go up, blood sugar goes down. When you take sugar from the brain, the brain gets severely fatigued (many of you readers will note this happening between 3 and 4 in the afternoon). Remember, progesterone helps stabilize blood sugar and often eliminates afternoon fatigue.

Another cause of her fatigue was depression. This was caused by a low progesterone level as well as internalization of anger. She also had asthma, which can produce a lowering of oxygen levels, contributing to fatigue.

A low thyroid level by itself can cause fatigue. She was on Claritin for allergies and Paxil for depression—side effects of these drugs include weakness and fatigue.

Why couldn't doctors help her? As I've said before, doctors are for the most part unaware of the pivotal role of hormones in sustaining health. They simply don't know how easy it is to help people like Rhonda. For me, turning Rhonda's health around was simple: We adjusted a couple of little things here and there. It's not hard to take care of patients. You just have to listen to them and be aware of how hormones affect the body.

Rhonda's brand of fatigue was something I would never have confused with chronic fatigue syndrome, which is a disease associated with fevers and swollen lymph glands. But I think many doctors misdiagnose people like Rhonda, treating them for chronic fatigue syndrome when what they actually have is a simple case of unbalanced hormones. You can see how people like Rhonda could be labeled as having chronic fatigue syndrome. The signs and symptoms are there, but the underlying causes are different.

DRUGS AND MORE DRUGS

This brings up another point I will make again and again in this book: the tendency of many members of the medical community to over-prescribe drugs as a consequence of misdiagnosing simple hormone imbalances. Besides the anti-depressant Paxil, Rhonda was also taking Claritin, prednisone, Prevacid and Synthroid. Each drug had one or more side effects, and Rhonda's body was spiraling out of control under the influence of all of these chemicals.

My first step with patients like Rhonda is to get them off of as many medications as possible while giving them progesterone to start the healing process. I would not have just stopped Paxil; I would have recommended that she start tapering off her use. I would have told her that progesterone would take away her asthma, so she could start weaning herself off her asthma medication, too.

Progesterone has a significant positive influence on asthma in both men and women. I suspect it is estrogen that creates asthma in many people. Keep in mind that men and women have the same hormones.

I had a male patient, 57 years old, who came to see me

because of weight concerns. He was on four medications for asthma. I told him that in three weeks he would be off all of his asthma medications. He said, "Doc, I've had asthma for 35 years and the Mayo Clinic prescribes my medications." I said, "Watch." In three weeks he came into my office, sat down and said, "Doc, you won't believe this...I'm off all of my medications for asthma!"

Progesterone treats asthma for two reasons—it blocks estrogen, a very common cause of asthma, and it breaks down into cortisone, which relieves asthma. Also, people with a lack of progesterone very commonly have hay fever. They discover that within two weeks of starting progesterone, all their hay fever and allergies are gone.

The prednisone Rhonda had been prescribed for her asthma was hurting her more than it was helping her. Prednisone has a lot of side effects. It can cause osteoporosis, cataracts, stomach ulcers and weight gain.

LOW THYROID

Doctors had prescribed Synthroid for Rhonda's low metabolism, but it actually had little effect. This is something we saw with Brenda J., too. She was also taking Synthroid but it wasn't helping with her thyroid problem.

Why her under active thyroid condition was missed was actually due to several factors. Before I go on, let me say that my goal is not to make endocrinologists out of my readers. (Endocrinologists are experts in the functions of the endocrine glands such as the pituitary and the thyroid.) But it is important to appreciate that the functioning of the body is very complex and for the most part it is regulated by the hormone system. If a doctor does not have a complete understanding of hormones, he or she will have a hard time trying to figure out how the body operates.

With that said, Rhonda had a condition called secondary hypothyroidism. This is caused by an insufficient amount of TSH being put out by the pituitary. Her free T3 level was below normal. Her pituitary should have been pouring out TSH to elevate this level, but it wasn't. A doctor only looking at TSH levels would fail to diagnose her condition. Correct thyroid testing would have easily picked this up. Her elevated cholesterol also pointed to a low thyroid.

OTHER BENEFITS OF PROGESTERONE

Rhonda had high blood pressure. Fifty percent of people with high blood pressure have it because they over-produce insulin. As I've mentioned before, hyperinsulinemia (too much insulin in the blood stream) is associated with low progesterone levels. Sometimes just reducing patients' insulin levels with progesterone relieves their high blood pressure.

Her depression was at least partly due to low progesterone. Progesterone is a natural anti-depressant, so women with low progesterone will commonly be depressed.

Rhonda was a wonderful candidate for progesterone. It had multiple benefits for her. Just by putting her on progesterone I was able to lower her insulin levels, eliminate her high-blood pressure, help her to begin losing weight, help relieve her depression and get rid of the asthma.

It's possible the progesterone helped with her acid reflux problem, too. Rhonda was on a drug called Prevacid that reduces acid secretion. By lowering insulin levels and reducing certain carbohydrates, you can cut down acid secretion, so the reflux would have gone away also. Adding digestive enzymes with each meal can also reduce acid reflux.

SUMMING UP

Getting Rhonda's life turned around was a simple matter of adding several hormones and eliminating the medications she was taking, along with their concomitant side effects.

In my initial interview with her, Rhonda indicated she was on a number of medications including thyroid, an antihistamine, an antidepressant, prednisone and a medication to prevent acid reflux. Although she was taking thyroid medication, she had all the classic symptoms of an under active thyroid: dry skin, nails that chipped easily, low body temperature, and so on. Like many people she was unable to convert the thyroid she was given into the active form, so she remained hypothyroid in spite of having been treated.

This, of course, contributed to her feeling tired all the time.

Rhonda was estrogen dominant, indicating low progesterone levels. This was the cause of her miscarriages, difficulty with conception, morning sickness, fibroid tumors, and endometriosis. Another symptom of low progesterone levels is hyperinsulinemia (high insulin levels). Insulin controls blood sugar: When insulin goes up, blood sugar goes down. When the brain doesn't get enough blood sugar, it falls asleep. This, too, contributed to her overall sense of fatigue.

Another factor causing fatigue was her depression. Some of her depression was related to suppressed anger, which manifested as fibromyalgia, a condition in which the body contracts its muscles even during sleep. Patients with this condition wake up stiff in the morning, often with pain and feeling as though they haven't had enough rest. Prolonged muscle tensing uses up energy, causing daytime fatigue.

Estrogen dominance and low progesterone levels also contributed to her developing allergies and asthma. She was placed on antihistamines, which unfortunately compounded her fatigue.

She was given prednisone for her asthma. Prednisone has the side effect of elevating sugar levels, leading to more insulin production, which added to Rhonda's hypoglycemia, a condition that results in feelings of fatigue.

She was prescribed the anti-depressant Paxil, which has its own list of multiple side effects, including weight gain, loss of libido and—you guessed it—fatigue. When you add up all of the fatigue-inducing chemicals she was both ingesting and producing within her own body, it's a wonder Rhonda was able to accomplish anything at all.

Again, my approach to this patient was simply to deal with the underlying causes rather than the symptoms of her fatigue. Adding progesterone eliminated her estrogen dominance and restored normal insulin levels. This in turn eliminated her asthma, part of her depression, her hypoglycemia and her allergies, allowing me to wean her off the fatigue-inducing medications prednisone and Paxil.

Now we're halfway home. The patient's got more control over her life, she's feeling better and as a result, she's not feeling so angry. Her fibromyalgia, with all the muscle tensing and the fatigue that comes from that, goes away. Adding T3, the thyroid hormone her body craves, gives her even more feelings of well-being, allowing her to lose weight and move even further away from depression.

THE FUEL TO KEEP FAMILIES RUNNING

Rhonda continues to do well with her weight and, more importantly, with her energy and ability to function within her family. I have had other patients who weren't so lucky. I have seen marriages flounder on the issue of fatigue. Without a high energy level it's almost impossible to be effective as a homemaker and mother.

When I read the statistics about the vast number of American women taking anti-depressants, I wonder how many of them would be better served having their metabolisms energized through the use of natural hormones. I would like to see more doctors who understand the role hormones play in creating and sustaining a normal zest for life—something that is everyone's birthright. Everyone should be able to benefit from the miracle of bio-identical hormones.

CHAPTER 5

MEDICATIONS THAT PREVENT WEIGHT LOSS

Many of the medications commonly prescribed by doctors today affect people's ability to manage their weight. Some of these effects are publicized and some aren't. For instance, most people taking Prozac know that it causes weight gain, and they make a conscious choice to sacrifice optimum weight management in order to get an improvement in their emotional outlook.

But the lipogenic (fat creating) effects of other medications aren't well known. People who take these medications may be struggling with their weight, unaware they're fighting a losing battle against a hidden enemy. These people should at least know what they are up against.

ANTI-DEPRESSANTS

Anti-depressants are a major source of weight gain for people. I suspect this happens in part because anti-depressants may elevate estrogen levels.

SSRIs (Selective Serotonin Reuptake Inhibitors) like Zoloft, Paxil, Effexor, Celexa, Lexapro and Prozac are particularly prone to causing weight gain. Some doctors prescribe these anti-depressants to help people *lose* weight by elevating their serotonin levels—serotonin is the neurotransmitter in the brain that takes away cravings. Those people who have a weight problem only because they crave certain foods can sometimes find a benefit in taking anti-depressants. But, for the most part, people on anti-depressants will gain weight.

The tricyclic anti-depressants like Elavil, Desipramine and Norpramin also cause weight gain.

A common phenomenon in our society is that people who are depressed about their weight start taking anti-depressants to help them with their depression. But then the anti-depressants cause further weight gain, making these people feel even worse about themselves. It's a vicious cycle.

In my experience, the only anti-depressant that possibly doesn't cause weight gain is Wellbutrin.

BETA-BLOCKERS

People taking beta-blockers are almost guaranteed to gain weight. Drugs like Lopressor, Atenolol, Ziac, and Inderal block adrenaline from entering the bloodstream. Adrenaline is what the body uses to stimulate the release of fat from the fat cells. If you can't get fat out of the fat cells, the muscles can't burn it.

Beta-blockers are also anti-thyroid drugs, as I mentioned in Chapter Three. One of the treatments for someone with an overactive thyroid is to give them a beta-blocker to quiet the thyroid down. It prevents the conversion of T4 into T3, something we learned about previously.

Ironically, the biggest prescribers of beta-blockers are cardiologists, who prescribe it because it decreases the workload of the heart. I call this an irony, because obesity is a major risk factor for heart disease. Therefore what they are prescribing to reduce the heart's work will ultimately give the heart more work—in the form of excess weight the patient will soon carry around.

Beta-blockers very quickly reach a point of diminishing returns for patients at risk for heart disease. The weight these patients gain cancels out many benefits the beta-blockers might have offered at the outset.

ESTROGEN

Perhaps the biggest impact on women's overall tendency to gain weight comes from estrogen. I say this because estrogen is one of the largest-selling drugs in the world, and it is prescribed to women throughout their lives, whether in the form of birth control pills in their youth or as part of Hormone Replacement Therapy after menopause. Estrogen is lipogenic—it creates fat—and this includes both natural and synthetic estrogen.

Women who still have their uterus are always prescribed a progestin along with any estrogen they are taking. This is because unopposed estrogen has been found to cause cancer of the uterus. The progestin most commonly prescribed is Provera, which helps protect the uterus from cancer. But progestins are also lipogenic, and like estrogen, produce cellulite and fat, and increase the risk of breast cancer.

Women who take Depo-Provera shots for birth control are practically guaranteed a 20 pound weight gain.

DIURETICS

Many people take diuretics for high blood pressure, and these medications can elevate blood sugar. Anything that elevates blood sugar will increase insulin production and, as I've said before, insulin is the fat-creating hormone.

ANTI-INFLAMMATORY DRUGS

Patients taking anti-inflammatory medication very often report an immediate weight gain. The weight gain caused by anti-inflammatory drugs is probably a result of fluid retention.

Statin drugs like Lipitor, Zocor, Pravachol, Mevacor, Lescol, and Crestor, etc. can also cause weight gain. This is because they lower coenzyme Q1O levels preventing the conversion of T4 (thyroxine) into T3 (liothyronine), the active thyroid hormone. Again, people concerned with weight want their thyroid to function as well as possible.

Interestingly, the most commonly prescribed drugs in this country all have the tendency to put on weight. Could this be contributing to the epidemic of obesity in this country? Could this be why people almost always have the tendency to put weight back on after they struggle to lose it? Could this be why some people cannot lose weight, no matter what they do?

CHAPTER 6

ROGER P. and MORBID OBESITY

Roger P., 47, arrived for his intake interview weighing 420 pounds. His pear-shaped body was the classic body type for someone pouring out excess estrogen along with too much insulin.

His hormone imbalance was accompanied by a host of other problems. He was reclusive, a drinker, and his body was in constant pain. As Roger tells his story, I hope to point the readers' attention toward his struggle against obesity, which created devastating physical and emotional havoc.

I've been fat my whole life. Being the fat kid in school made me an outcast. When you're always on the outside looking in, your level of caring declines. I felt that everything and everyone was against me and I was an angry kid.

Not only was I fat but I was weird looking, too. I carried all my weight in my hips and thighs, like a woman. I was one of those obese people who seem to be not a "he" or a "she" but an "it." I looked like two different people stuck together.

In my line of work, which is designing and building binary data systems, I'm able to work solo as a contract employee. I always chose to work from home, going in for meetings as infrequently as possible. I fashioned my career to allow for maximum reclusiveness.

I was always ashamed and embarrassed. Whenever I went out to eat I would find the darkest, most secluded corner in the restaurant to hide out in. Clothes were a problem, too. For years' I wore bib overalls, the monster size. I couldn't button them all the way up on the sides.

And I lived in fear of children. Children would see me in public and pipe up with something totally humiliating. I started scheduling my visits to the market for the middle of the night just to avoid being humiliated by little kids.

In the midst of all of this humiliation, I had a strong feeling that this obesity was not my fault. I would keep going to doctors to try and get some help. Normally their response, after they'd taken my money, was to say, "Go home, kid, and quit eating so much." I would tell them, "I don't eat that much," and I didn't, I never have. You and I could eat the same exact meal and you'd be unaffected, but I'd wake up the next morning and my pants wouldn't fit. But every doctor I tried to get help from told me that although I probably didn't think I was a huge eater, in reality I was. They made me feel like a liar. Some of them gave me amphetamines.

At age 23 I started getting leg pains, and then later on I developed full body cramps. I was cramping all the time, having night sweats and weird vision problems. None of the doctors I went to had any solutions for me. These problems were variously misdiagnosed as gout, pseudo-gout, tendonitis and a bunch of other things.

My life was miserable. I'd do my work, come home, drink a six-pack of beer and a half bottle of Tequila every night and go to sleep and get up and do the whole thing over again. One night a friend infuriated me on the phone by telling me I was like some little old lady with her two dogs and no life. It sent me off the scale. I yelled at her. But I thought about it all night, and the next day I realized that she had only described me as I really was.

I had heard Dr. Platt talking about weight loss on the radio. The day after the fight with my friend I went to see him. He sat me down and talked to me for over an hour. He wanted to know everything about my family history and my life. After my initial visit he put me on progesterone and DHEA and started me on the diet. Right away I started losing weight.

About three months into the program I had a real bad flare-up in my knee, hip and in-between; it felt like having hot steel shoved up your leg. I tried a chiropractor and then a sports medicine specialist, but they didn't help. Finally I thought, "what the heck; I'll ask Dr. Platt about it."

I was totally shocked by his reaction. "Look, I'm your physician and I'm treating you," he said. "I want to know everything that's happening to you." I found that such a strange attitude for a doctor.

He added testosterone and thyroid to my medications, and changed the type of DHEA I was taking. That same day he diagnosed my fibromyalgia, which is the pain in my leg that had been misdiagnosed by so many doctors. About three days later I felt as though I'd come out of a fog. It's hard to describe. I had been there so long I didn't know I was there. I had an amazing change, a new clarity of thought. It was startling.

And I was pain-free for the first time in 24 years. Strange things started happening to me physically at this point. All my life I've been kind of a big, white, farm-boy-looking guy without any muscle definition at all. Now I've developed all this muscle definition. I'm much stronger. I used to sleep eight or ten hours a day and then sit all day without wanting to do anything. Now I sleep about four hours a night and I'm never tired. Life is good.

I weigh 195 pounds. It's the first time I've been less than 200 pounds since I was 12 years old. My brain hasn't kept up with my body and my biggest challenges now are social and psychological. I'd say socially I'm probably at a junior high school grade level because I've never participated in society outside of work.

People sometimes ask me if I'm bitter about all the years when I was looking for help and doors were being shut in my face. But I'm not. They were blessings and gifts even though they were painful. I'm pretty happy with who I am now.

THE PAIN OF MORBID OBESITY

To me, Roger P's case highlights the pivotal problem with the way medicine is practiced today.

As I've said before, doctors don't have the one hour it takes to listen to their patients any more. For years Roger went from doctor to doctor about his weight problem, telling them that he didn't overeat and asking for help. But they didn't listen to him. They dismissed him.

And they didn't *observe* him. They didn't *look* at him. It was so obvious from the distribution of his fat that there was something more than an eating problem going on. He *had* to have a hormone problem—it was obvious. It's amazing to me that so many doctors were blind to it.

When I went through medical school, we had a course called "Physical Diagnosis," and it was fascinating. We learned about an array of physical signs, many of them very subtle, that you could observe in a patient to pick up information about what might be going on inside their bodies. It was a kind of visual detective work. It kept you attuned to what you were really seeing when you looked at your patient.

I doubt that they even teach this course any more. The medical profession has become so fixated on technology that simple, first-person observation has ceased to have much value to many doctors.

TWO STEPS FORWARD—ONE STEP BACK

This may sound strange, but I often feel that a major setback in medicine has been the development of blood tests. In the old days—going back 100 to 200 years ago—the only thing doctors had to rely on was talking to their patients and observing them. (In the really early days they didn't even have stethoscopes. They'd roll up a piece of paper and listen to people's hearts through that.) Today doctors have blood tests to fall back on, and the statistical "hard facts" of blood tests seem to be reassuring to them. They'd rather treat the blood test than look at the patient and find out what's actually going on. With every technological advance, it seems as though doctors recede further and further from direct contact with their patients.

Roger P. was a patient who was obviously crying out for help, and nobody would give it to him. He was just about suicidal when he came to me. Looking at him, at the way he stored fat in the abdomen and buttocks, it was obvious to me that his body produced too much insulin and estrogen. So I put him on progesterone right away. He went on the diet, and I eventually added other hormones to help him with his metabolism and muscle mass.

THE ROAD HOME

As he lost weight, Roger's anger melted away too, and that helped to mitigate his fibromyalgia. This man had been furious for practically all of his 47 years. He'd been a fat child, and we all know how cruel children are to the fat kids at school. As an adult he carried this humiliation with him, becoming a recluse and living a life of quiet desperation. The suppressed anger he felt must have been crushing.

Once he finally got help at our office, once he talked to a doctor who confirmed that he was *not* overeating and he was *not* the cause of his own disfigurement, his gratitude knew no bounds. Today Roger will tell anyone who will listen that he'd walk through fire for me or anyone in my office.

If you saw Roger today, you would never know this man had once been morbidly obese. He looks like a normal person and his entire life has been transformed. And it was so simple. It was just a matter of getting his hormones in balance and getting him to eat in a way that would force his body to burn fat.

THE INFORMATION IS AVAILABLE

The sad thing is that what I'm doing for people like Roger is based on information that's available to any doctor who wants to avail himself or herself of it. This is not secret information.

The other day I saw an ad in the newspaper for "An Amazing Weight Loss Discovery." It was a pill that "caused the body to get rid of fat in three different ways," and you didn't have to change anything in your lifestyle, you could still continue to eat everything, you wouldn't have to exercise and the fat would just come right off, etc., etc., etc...

I'm sure you've seen such ads and scoffed at their disingenuousness. These ads all have little disclaimers way down at the bottom of the page, usually next to some before-and-after photos, saying "Results not typical." Well, if these aren't the typical results, then why buy the pills? They typically don't work! It says so right there in the ad!

I'm being a bit facetious here, but it's for a good reason. I'm trying to drive home the point that as a society we tolerate all kinds of ridiculous misinformation about weight loss, while real information that could actually help people goes unheeded.

It's my hope that people suffering from morbid obesity will take this book into their doctors' offices and demand the simple, inexpensive solutions to their plight that they deserve.

THE FINAL CHAPTER

At the time Roger, aged 47, walked into my office, he told me he had never had a date in his life. He started on the program, lost weight, got down to a size 32 waist, eliminated his fibromyalgia, started dating, got engaged…and is now happily married.

It is truly miraculous what a little natural hormone balance can accomplish.

CHAPTER 7

THE ROLE OF EXERCISE IN WEIGHT MANAGEMENT

I am a big fan of physical exercise. As a weight management tool it has untold advantages.

During the weight loss phase of my weight management system, I recommend physical exercise as a way to help my patients burn fat more quickly. This is the phase when the substances the muscles normally oxidize for energy—glycogen and sugar—have been removed, leaving the body no choice except to burn fat. In this phase every movement of the body burns fat. Any *extra* movement the body gets, in the form of walking, lifting weights, swimming—any kind of physical activity—simply speeds up the fat-burning process.

My patients who are able to exercise during this period—
that is, patients who are in good health, without pain and not
so obese that movement is difficult for them—report that
exercise in this phase is extremely satisfying. It helps their
mood, helps them relax and get better sleep, increases mental
alertness, and ultimately adds to their self-esteem and self-
confidence. And as the pounds come off they feel rewarded for
their efforts.

For people who haven't exercised in a long time—and that
includes many obese people who find exercise exhausting—I
recommend they spend the first week of the weight loss program walking (or doing very light, low-impact aerobic activity) for 15 to 30 minutes, 3 times a week.

By the second month I recommend they follow the same
schedule but walk a bit faster.

Of course, if they feel motivated to exercise more often, I
would never stop them. But I recommend they keep it pleas-
ant. If exercise starts to become a chore they should back off.
What they want to do here is to establish a habit they can keep
up over the long haul, even when they've reached their ideal
weight (*especially* when they've reached their ideal weight).
People will usually stop doing something that's unpleasant. If
they exercise only out of a sense of duty, without a pleasurable
payoff, they won't be able to make exercise a lifetime habit.

FORGET CALORIES

Another piece of advice I give is not to think about exercise as
burning calories. We have been so brainwashed by this count-
ing-calories approach to weight management in our society. It's
reached the point where people see exercise in a strictly
mechanical way, as something they reluctantly do to counter-
act the effects of eating.

What a negative concept! Exercise can be delightful when you find the type of movement that's right for you. We're meant to move our bodies around in this world. It's part of the pleasure of living.

Exercise should not be seen as an obligation. It is pleasurable in its own right, part of an enjoyable and active life. It does much more than burn calories—it stimulates all kinds of healthful reactions in the body, including the production of neurotransmitters (such as endorphins) that create feelings of well-being and pleasure. If we think about all the subtle, wonderful things our bodies are doing while we are walking, swimming or whatever, exercise will take on a whole new dimension.

BOTH ANAEROBIC AND AEROBIC

Both anaerobic exercise (such as weight lifting) and aerobic exercise (such as walking) is fruitful during the weight loss phase.

Anaerobic exercise, which adds muscle mass, increases the body's ability to burn fat. It adds muscle tissue—that is, fat-burning tissue—which speeds up the fat-burning process. Aerobic exercise is good for the heart, and it also gradually brings the metabolism to a higher level. I recommend that my patients start increasing their aerobic workouts in the second month of the program, working at 60 percent to 70 percent of their maximum heart rate for at least 20 minutes, 3 times a week, with a 5 minute warm-up and a 5 minute cool-down.

ESSENTIAL FOR WEIGHT MAINTENANCE

During the second part of the weight management system, the maintenance phase, exercise is the single most important factor in maintaining a stable weight. This is particularly true for those who want to keep high-glycemic carbohydrates in their meal plans, such as bread, potatoes, cereal, etc. The body always prioritizes replacing glycogen (sugar) into muscle tissue. This is a survival mechanism. The body wants to ensure that muscles always have enough energy. If you take in more sugar than your muscles require, the excess will be stored in your fat cells.

The more you exercise, the more glycogen you burn, and the more of your carbohydrate intake goes into muscle instead of being stored as fat. When you are at your ideal weight, it is easy to stay there as long as you are getting enough exercise.

PUTTING EXERCISE INTO PERSPECTIVE

In order to burn off one pound of fat, there has to be a 3500 calorie deficit. The amount of exercise required for this would be equal to going out and running 35 miles. If you've ever been on a treadmill and pushed the calorie counter at the end it might register about 140 calories or up to 350 if you've struggled. No where near the 3500 calories required to lose one pound. You would have to stay on the treadmill for 7 1/2 hours going 4 mph to lose one pound.

A famous exercise guru seen on infomercials exhorting people to exercise has himself undergone gastric bypass surgery. A famous actress—turned weight loss guru has herself only been able to get rid of fat via liposuction (this is not recommended for weight loss).

In other words, exercise enhances weight loss but only in conjunction with the correct meal plan, hormone balance and getting off of certain medications, etc.

People who are 100-200 pounds or more over-weight, do not even have to exercise. Every time they walk, this represents a weight-bearing exercise. After they have lost a *significant* amount, then they can start on a program.

Let me again stress that the key to losing weight is eating correctly, not exercise. If you are exercising, you must insure that the body is getting enough fuel, otherwise it will convert to fat-storing rather than fat-burning.

I have had patients who have lived on 800 calories a day, exercised 4 hours a day and could not lose an ounce.

In the last chapter I will address weight loss.

CHAPTER 8

LOUIS R. and ADULT-ONSET DIABETES

Louis R. is a successful and contented 60-year-old who's struggled with weight all his life. When I took his family history, it became clear that his weight problem was genetic. Everyone in his family—mother, father, aunts, uncles, grandparents—was "heavyset."

When we talked about his goals, Louis emphasized that he was bound and determined not to "let himself go" at age 60, the way many of his family members had done.

When his treatment is completed, Louis can be assured he'll be able to control his weight without dieting. He'll also be able to manage his adult-onset diabetes without the use of medication.

I am a Type II diabetic. My diabetes started in middle age, but even before that I'd always experienced problems with my weight. At six different times in my life I've been 40 pounds overweight, and I've dieted to lose those 40 pounds. Each time I was successful in losing the weight but over time those same 40 pounds reappeared. I have done Weight Watchers, I used Diet Center twice, and I've gone the Nutra System route and others. Each of these diets was effective. The pounds just flew off but psychologically I was about four feet off of the ground at all times. Either that or I was unbearably fatigued. My whole family is predisposed to being heavy. My father was a little shorter than me and at one time weighed about 240 pounds. My paternal grandmother was about six feet tall and a very big woman who weighed about 230 pounds. When my late sister was diagnosed with colon cancer she weighed 290 pounds. My maternal grandfather was large, as was my maternal grandmother.

So I'm from sturdy big stock and I'm never going to be one of those men who weigh 165 pounds. I know that. Once I dieted my way down to 168 pounds but I looked horrible. People were asking me what disease I had I was so gaunt. Today my goal is more realistic. I want to reach 185 pounds and stay there for the rest of my life. My other goal is to control my diabetes with diet and exercise.

When my mother turned 60, she told me, she just wanted to be a fat old lady. She just let everything go. When she died she was 5'2" and weighed about 240 pounds. I turned 60 last year and I decided I do not want to be like my mother. I'm going in the opposite direction. I want to slim down and build some muscle and remain attractive.

I have to say up front that when I first visited Dr. Platt, I walked into his office with an attitude of skepticism. Not because of all the diets I'd gone on, but because I have an insider's knowledge of medical scams. For 20 years my career consisted of marketing and selling pharmaceutical products. I know what pharmaceutical companies will stoop to in order to turn a profit. I lost my innocence about medicine long ago and I'm always on the lookout for someone trying to turn an easy buck.

But once I spoke to Dr. Platt I was relieved. From the way he talked, I realized he wasn't just promoting products. What he said about why people hang onto weight and why their bodies hate to lose fat, made sense. There was none of the jargon and medical babble that tends to cluster around trendy medical scams.

Platt's office staff has also been very supportive and they communicate a sense of being genuinely interested in everyone who comes in there. The whole atmosphere is wonderful. They're not punitive when you don't meet your goals as expected.

As far as the process of losing weight is concerned, it's been virtually painless. The diet itself is easy to follow. I'm a fruit freak and that's been the most difficult thing to give up, but I realize that I will be able to go back to fruit later in the process; it's not something I have to give up for the rest of my life. Once I've lost the weight I want to lose, the fruit will be re-introduced. In the short term, trust me, if that's all I have to give up, that's fine.

There was a brief period when I was losing weight but not feeling very energetic. I went in to see one of the nutritional counselors and was recommended a multi-mineral. It was my thought, knowing just enough about medicine to be dangerous, that perhaps I should be taking potassium. I know diets can be potassium-depleting. But the counselor said not only to do potassium, but to take a multi-mineral as well. Sure enough, my energy returned and I started feeling absolutely great. It made me wonder whether I'd been lacking in some mineral or other for many years.

During my very first interview with Dr. Platt it came out that my sister died of colon cancer, and now one of her daughters has colon cancer. Also, my mother had a mastectomy when she was 38. Dr. Platt was very interested in this. It's one of the reasons why he placed me on progesterone, which is erroneously thought of as a female hormone. But according to him, progesterone will protect me from the excess estrogen

I'm putting out. He knew that was true even before he did my blood work, just from my family medical history.

I was also started on testosterone and the amounts were very carefully monitored by Dr. Platt's office. It certainly helped with my libido (interest in sex). According to the blood work my DHEA is that of a 30-year-old. Dr. Platt wanted to know if anyone in my family had lived a long time. My grandfather was almost 90 and my mother was almost 90 when she died.

Dr. Platt also thought my thyroid was not putting out as much hormone as it should, so he has me on a couple of thyroid medications. This makes a difference. I've noticed since I've been on this diet that I don't get that late afternoon letdown I used to get. I think that's due to the thyroid medications, and the progesterone, which Dr. Platt states is stabilizing my blood sugar.

So far I've lost 32 pounds, and I've weaned myself off one of my medications for diabetes. As we go along we're fine-tuning my medications. It seems to be a rather sensible approach. I'm very pleased with the results.

DIABETES AND INSULIN

Roger has a strong family history of both obesity and adult-onset diabetes. This means everyone in his family overproduces insulin, and insulin is the hormone that creates fat.

A simple way of thinking about insulin is to understand that insulin will take any sugar that the body's not using and store it primarily in the fat cells. Once the sugar is absorbed into the fat cells it is converted into fat. People have a limited number of fat cells, which can only contain a limited amount of fat. As these cells fill up with fat, it gets harder for insulin to get the sugar into them. This is called 'insulin resistance.' The body responds to this by producing even more insulin. This is called 'hyperinsulinemia'. Insulin not only creates fat, it prevents fat from getting out of the fat cells—it is a fat-storing hormone.

One can easily see that if you have too much insulin, you are going to have a weight problem.

Eventually the fat cells get completely filled up and sugar can no longer get into the fat cells—it builds up in the blood stream and a patient is told he or she has diabetes. Doctors approach diabetes like it is a disease of high blood sugar when, actually, it is frequently a disease of too much insulin.

So patients are given medications to stimulate the pancreas to make even more insulin—this extra insulin literally pushes the sugar into the fat cells creating even more weight gain.

The exception to this is the medication Glucophage, which goes by the generic name metformin. This medication does not actually lower blood sugar. It acts by increasing the sensitivity of tissues in the body to insulin, leading to a lowering of insulin levels. Needless to say, I do not wean people off this particular diabetic medication. I will be devoting a special chapter to weight loss in diabetics.

There are many patients with Type II diabetes (adult-onset) who wind up on insulin. Keep in mind that probably 90 percent of people with adult-onset diabetes already have too much insulin to begin with. Very often, placing patients on insulin exacerbates their problem. This is because insulin is not only promoting the movement of sugar into fat cells; it is also preventing the release of fat because it is a fat-storing hormone.

HYPOGLYCEMIA AND INSULIN

If my patients are having hypoglycemic reactions, usually manifested by afternoon fatigue, sleepiness after eating, sleepiness while in a car, either as the driver or as a passenger, this tells me that they are over-producing insulin, irrespective of blood sugar levels. It's becoming fairly well accepted that insulin is the main cause of weight problems. It is the hormone that not only creates fat, but sits there and prevents the release of fat from the fat cells—it is the ideal fat-storing hormone.

I will be discussing insulin in the Chapter on Permanent Weight Loss, but at this point I would like to address two key factors with regard to Louis.

In my opinion, there is one major cause for hyperinsulinemia (too much insulin)—too little progesterone. Louis' family history was classic for this condition, which underlines the importance of talking to your patients. Much information can be gleaned from a family history. In the first place, the prevalence of diabetes was suggestive of Syndrome X, the form of hyperinsulinemia associated with high triglyceride levels and low HDL cholesterol. In addition, the strong family history of estrogen-related cancers again suggested low progesterone levels. Again, bio-identical progesterone most likely prevents every cancer caused by estrogen.

HORMONAL INFLUENCES

Louis had significant hormone problems. His family history was consistent with estrogen dominance and low progesterone levels. The history of colon cancer and breast cancer among the women in his family was related to estrogen. The low progesterone led to problems with hyperinsulinemia, with resultant obesity.

Blood tests indicated that he had low levels of testosterone. This too is a hormone that lowers insulin levels, just like progesterone. Testosterone is probably the most important hormone to replace in a male, for multiple reasons. It treats and prevents osteoporosis (fractured hips are associated with a 25 percent mortality rate in men). It helps keep the heart healthy: the heart muscle has more testosterone receptor sites than any other muscle. That means the heart uses more testosterone than any other organ. Testosterone is now being used to treat congestive heart failure in men. A man cannot build muscle without testosterone. This hormone prevents Alzheimer's disease and a man will not have the ability to perform sexually with low levels of testosterone. It has been found that many men (and women) have very low levels of testosterone after a heart attack. Could it be a contributing factor?

DIABETES AND WEIGHT MANAGEMENT

Louis will probably have to restrict the carbohydrates in his diet for the rest of his life. Making Louis aware of how his metabolism works—how sugar and insulin throw his energy levels out of whack, and how he can use protein to stabilize his system—has made all the difference. With his hormones balanced and with a conscious attitude toward his diet, Louis is able to manage his weight and avoid the pitfalls of diabetes.

We have a nationwide epidemic of obesity and type II diabetes. Both of these conditions are strictly hormonal problems. Understanding this connection again allows one to appreciate the miraculous benefits of restoring hormonal balance with bio-identical hormones.

CHAPTER 9

GREG C. and PSYCHOGENIC MEDICATION

When Greg C. walked into my office I saw a handsome 32-year-old whose body had become distorted by weight gain. He talked earnestly and honestly about a recent nervous breakdown and the five powerful psychogenic drugs—almost all of them lipogenic (causing the body to store fat)—doctors said he needed for mental balance. I want him to tell his story for the benefit of the millions of people taking antidepressants and other psychogenic drugs who could live normal, happy lives if their hormones were balanced.

I've always been a high achiever. I set goals for myself and then I pursue them with everything I've got. For a long time this worked well for me. My achievements were pleasing to my parents who gave me a lot of approval and made me want to achieve even more. My father was very successful financially at a young age and placed a lot of value on worldly status and possessions. So did my mother and, of course, so did I.

By my mid-20s I was making a lot of money working in the hospitality business in Las Vegas. I had a responsible job at Caesar's Palace and I gave it everything I had, so much so that I was losing my balance. I worked so much that I stopped doing very much of anything else. Las Vegas is a 24-hour-a-day, 365-days-a-year place, a city that never sleeps, and demands are made on you constantly to keep the machinery running. I would always go the extra mile to troubleshoot an emergency, accommodate unexpected guests…whatever came up.

Somehow amidst all this work I did manage to meet a woman I wanted to spend my life with. Stephanie and I married when I was 30 and she got pregnant soon afterwards. This added even more responsibility, and although I didn't understand it then I began showing signs of nervous exhaustion.

I began to lose my appetite. I'm a wonderful cook—I went to school to become a chef early in my life and every day after work I'd come home and cook a healthy meal for my wife while she was pregnant but I found I couldn't eat. After the baby was born—he's a boy—I cooked for each of them, the kinds of nutritious meals I felt they should have, but again I couldn't eat the food I cooked. I'd have a piece of toast or something. For someone going at break neck speed the way I was, this wasn't good. I wasn't taking care of myself.

You see, I had this Superman complex where I felt I had to take care of everyone and everything. I never told my wife how scared I was of failing, because that wouldn't be taking care of her. I hid my insecurities and just pushed myself.

Often I'd go back to work after dinner. If my wife protested I'd make up a story about some emergency that had come up. The truth was I felt I had to do more just to keep up. It's a mindset. I felt things would fall apart if I didn't hurry up and do more.

At a certain point this became an issue for me and Stephanie, and we saw a counselor who suggested I work in a less stressful environment. I found a job at the Las Vegas Convention and Visitors' Authority, thinking it would allow me more time for a normal life. But just the opposite happened. I became even more stressed and worked even longer hours. Even with my son at home I couldn't tear myself away from work.

Stephanie insisted I see a psychiatrist about my workaholic attitude. I began seeing a woman who diagnosed me as bipolar and gave me four strong medications to even out my highs and lows. I began talk therapy as well.

Looking back, I probably should have gotten a second opinion from another psychiatrist. The talk therapy only dealt with my euphoria and my depression. We never talked about the underlying problems that were driving me. I began getting worse and worse. I felt so much responsibility that I couldn't handle it. There was nothing in my life that felt comfortable and grounded. I felt anxious all the time; I couldn't sleep or eat.

At one point I threatened to drive to Hoover Dam and jump. Stephanie got on her knees and cried and begged me to get some real help. There is a psychiatric hospital in Connecticut my family knows about and they offered to send me there. By now I'd lost my job. I knew that if I wanted to get my life on track I'd have to get more help.

So I spent the summer in Connecticut, getting a lot of individual counseling and group therapy, too. Stephanie went to Chicago with our son to stay with her parents. We lost our house. Stephanie is now in Chicago and we are both praying for reconciliation and a chance to start life over together.

In Connecticut they added lithium to the drugs I was taking, bringing the number to five. These were all very strong drugs, including Effexor, Paxil and Depakote. I didn't like the way I felt on the drugs. They made me drowsy and blurred my thinking.

Another side effect was weight gain. I went from my habitual 165 pounds (I'm 6 feet tall) up to 215.

When I left the psychiatric hospital, I came to the desert to stay with my mother. Today I'm under the care of a psychiatrist, going through a healing process. When I told a friend about how uncomfortable I felt weighing 215, he recommended I see Dr. Platt.

Initially I went just for the weight loss, but I have received so much more from my treatment. The great miracle is that not only have I gone back to my usual weight, I've been able to wean myself off all the drugs I was on.

My intake interview with Dr. Platt made me feel very comfortable. When I told him about all the drugs 1 was taking he told me I was over-medicated, and that if I followed his hormone treatment and his diet I would be able to wean myself off the drugs. I told my psychiatrist about Dr. Platt and he was open to the idea of helping the weaning process along as long as I continued in therapy with him and continued to examine the issues that got me into trouble in the first place.

I started Dr. Platt's treatment in January and set myself the goal of being drug-free and the proper weight by the end of March. I reached my goal by early March, and today feel absolutely fantastic. I feel so lucid and my thought processes are so clear compared to how I felt on the drugs.

I'm continuing in therapy and applying for jobs in various industries such as banking and insurance, more conventional industries where the hours are normal. I don't want to be in the hospitality business any more.

While I'm waiting for a job to come through, I'm delivering newspapers at night. It's something I never could have imagined myself doing at the age of 32. But it gives me time to think about what I want for my future, and I see the moon and stars every night and watch the sun rise every morning. It's a humbling experience, but it's also a rebirth. I feel the foundation of my house has been properly poured this time. I've gotten so much help with my world-view, both from my psychiatrist and Dr. Platt, who encourages me to approach life as an enjoyable journey. I'm thinking in a way I've never thought before. I used to have so much fear that I was never going to amount to anything in life. Now I know that if I stay balanced I will have an impact on the lives of my loved ones and hopefully my community, and that's all I want.

THE DANGERS OF PSYCHOTROPHIC MEDICATION

This patient presents a classic example of how medications can contribute to a person's problems instead of helping them.

When I look at patients, my approach is always to look for the underlying causes of their problems. I can't just look at problems without seeing the entire person. Greg came to me for weight loss but I would not treat him as a straightforward weight management patient without addressing these five incredibly powerful drugs he was taking. I knew that even if I were to get him down to his ideal weight, those drugs would eventually bring him right back to where he was. So I addressed the psychogenic drugs first.

Although I'm not a psychiatrist, I found the diagnosis of bipolar disorder suspicious. That's a very specific disorder—one that tends to be over-diagnosed, by the way. I didn't believe that Greg was really suffering from that malady. Since I know that hormones have a tremendous impact on the neurotransmitters in the brain, I decided to go on the working theory that Greg, like many people, was being diagnosed with something very serious when in fact he was probably just suffering from unbalanced hormones.

Whatever Greg's psychological difficulties were, I knew that with the right hormones he could get relief from his symptoms. I told Greg that my goal for him was to get him off his drugs and to get his hormones in balance. He was delighted with that, since he felt foggy and uncomfortable on them.

Fortunately, Greg's psychiatrist was open to the idea of weaning him off of these powerful drugs. It was his feeling that Greg's nervous breakdown was an extreme stress reaction, not a symptom of bipolar disorder, and that if Greg could address his issues in talk therapy he could eventually go back to living a normal, drug-free life.

INSURANCE HAPPENS

Greg initially came to me because of a concern about weight. This problem was caused by a combination of too much insulin plus the medications he was on. Since most of Greg's weight had settled in around his abdomen, I knew I was dealing with someone who was overproducing insulin. I started him on natural progesterone right away. I did this for four reasons:

- Progesterone reduces insulin

- Progesterone regulates blood sugar levels

- Progesterone is wonderful for brain tissue (as I've mentioned before, progesterone levels are 20 times higher in brain tissue than anywhere else)

- Progesterone is a natural anti-depressant

Between progesterone and the meal plan, Greg began losing weight right away. With his psychiatrist's help, he slowly reduced the amount of Paxil, Effexor, Depakote and Lithium he was taking. As he continuously lowered the dosages of those lipogenic medications, his weight loss speeded up.

He got into a positive feedback loop whereby he liked the way he was looking, which led to feeling better about himself and making faster progress in talk therapy, which led to further success with his weight management program, and so on. As the weeks went by you could see the transformation.

Eventually Greg returned to being the person he'd been before he'd started the medications, minus the driven, workaholic overlay. Today he's a very energetic, forward-looking person with a lot to live for.

Greg will eventually be reunited with his wife and child. With the help of hormones, he'll be able to live a balanced life that he truly enjoys. In addition, he is now acutely aware of the importance of balancing his son's hormones and his wife's hormones.

Greg's problems were strictly hormonal: too much adrenalin, too much insulin, too much cortisol, and too little progesterone. Putting them back into balance gave him the "miracle" he was looking for.

THE UNDERLYING PROBLEM

Greg is a classic example of the powerful effect hormones have on our health. He also illustrates why it is so important to understand the background of your patients.

When I first talked with Greg, it was immediately apparent to me that he had classic ADHD (attention deficit hyperactivity disorder). Adults with this problem frequently become workaholics and type A personalities. These people thrive on adrenalin because they are persistently hypoglycemic.

They start out with low progesterone levels, leading to the over-production of insulin. This leads to hypoglycemia and to an outpouring of adrenalin to bring sugar levels up.

This was Greg's underlying metabolic state. When he began working in Las Vegas, the new element of stress was added.

Now his adrenal glands were not only over-producing

adrenalin, but were also over-producing cortisol (this will be addressed in an upcoming chapter). The cortisol raised sugar levels, leading to even more insulin production. This led to more hypoglycemia, which led to more adrenalin. He lost his appetite because of the high levels of adrenalin, leading to a body starved for fuel, which created even more stress.

He did not have bi-polar disorder; he just had a major hormonal imbalance. One can readily see why people missing certain hormones can wind up with many psychological conditions that can be treated in a more effective manner than using drugs.

I will be addressing ADD/ADHD in a future chapter.

CHAPTER 10

DHEA, STRESS and PROSTATE CANCER

One hormone I've given only passing mention to so far is DHEA. It's a very important hormone, one whose full range of effects hasn't yet been plumbed by medical science. But we know enough about DHEA to know it is absolutely essential for optimal health.

DHEA is produced mainly by the adrenal glands, but also by the gonads, the brain and the skin, and at one stage it is the most abundant steroid hormone in the body. Since the 1980s there have been many research papers published indicating that DHEA has multiple healthful functions in the body. It prevents heart disease and prostate cancer in men, osteoporosis and breast cancer in women.

DHEA levels decline in a straight line as we age. This hormone begins to appear in our bodies at age 6, peaks during the 20's, is at 50 percent level at age 40, and between the ages of 60 and 80 declines to between 20 percent and 10 percent of peak levels. This definitive decrease is not seen with other hormones and, because of this, some believe that many of the manifestations of aging are caused by deficiencies of DHEA.

Administration of DHEA is associated with a remarkable increase in perceived physical and psychological well-being. These benefits are noticed after four months of therapy. People report increased energy, better sleep, a significant improvement in sexuality and in mood, along with a better ability to handle stress. DHEA has been shown to enhance memory and mental acuity and to decrease depression. Administration of DHEA helps to boost the immune system, improves chronic fatigue syndrome, helps to reduce body fat, and improves autoimmune diseases such as lupus, ulcerative colitis and rheumatoid arthritis.

People with high levels of DHEA have lower incidences of Alzheimer's and Parkinson's disease. A low DHEA level is felt by some to be the most significant biological marker for breast cancer in premenopausal women.

DHEA AND STRESS

People who live with a lot of stress start to show lowered DHEA levels after a certain amount of time. Their adrenal glands become exhausted, and since the adrenal glands produce DHEA, their DHEA goes way down. Airline pilots, for instance, whose days consist of meeting strict schedules despite unpredictable weather, performing numerous take-offs and landings (landings often involve split-second timing and near misses), and other stressful situations, often show up in my office with little or no DHEA on their hormone panels.

It's well known that pilots report unusually high levels of prostate cancer. Many of them theorize that this might be caused by the radiation they are constantly exposed to flying at high altitudes. But it's my theory that lack of DHEA may contribute to the problem. The other cause is lack of progesterone.

Progesterone also diminishes in people who live under constant stress. The most dramatic example of this is seen in women living in abusive situations. They have almost no DHEA on their hormone panels, and they tend to show all the signs of estrogen dominance as well. Living in constant fear depletes both DHEA and progesterone.

Women can get cancer of the uterus from estrogen dominance. When I treat a woman living in an abusive situation I will invariably prescribe both DHEA and progesterone.

PROGESTERONE THERAPY FOR MEN

It is important to keep in mind that men and women produce identical hormones, although in different amounts. Some doctors do not consider progesterone to be a male hormone (it is) and some are not aware that men produce estrogen (they do).

I prescribe progesterone to most of my male patients over 50 for a number of reasons. One is that I suspect that it prevents prostate cancer. I cannot point to studies that show this, but it is logical. As men approach their andropause (the male menopause, starting around age 50), their progesterone levels drop and their estrogen levels start rising.

This is also about the time that prostate cancer becomes a risk. The only known cause for cancer of the uterus is estrogen.

The prostate is derived embryologically from the exact tissue that the uterus comes from. So if estrogen causes uterine cancer, why wouldn't it be causing prostate cancer? Men start having very high levels of estradiol, the strongest estrogen, by the time they reach 60. They are no longer producing progesterone to protect them from all of this estrogen. And this is the moment in men's lives when prostate cancer becomes more frequent.

If estrogen causes six different cancers in women, why wouldn't it be up to no good in men as well? Not only cancer of the prostate but cancer of the colon could also be caused by excess estrogen in men's bodies.

If estrogen is indeed the cause of cancer of the prostate, the whole approach to treatment would have to change. Right now testosterone is thought to cause cancer of the prostate. Everything is done to eliminate testosterone in men who show symptoms of prostate cancer. Estrogen is at times given to treat prostate cancer. Could this be contributing to the death rate?

Could estrogen be the culprit in the epidemic of prostate cancer deaths in our society? It's worth considering. And it wouldn't hurt to look into changing some standard treatments. It's very possible that the way we treat prostate cancer today is actually doing more harm than good. It is strongly recommended that doctors start looking at estradiol levels in men. Please refer to the chapter on the andropause for advice on lowering estradiol levels.

THOUGHTS ON PROSTATE CANCER

Most men, if they live long enough, will develop prostate cancer. But only 7% of these cancers spread, so theoretically, 93% of men will die with prostate cancer rather than from it.

So let's say a man has an elevated PSA—a possible indication of cancer. He is whisked off to a urologist who promptly sticks a needle in his prostate (the standard of medical practice) to evaluate the high PSA. There is a good chance he might hit an area of cancer because of the multiple biopsies being taken. But is it possible that the cancer, which only had a 7% chance of getting out of the prostate, is now able to get into the blood stream and this is how it spreads?

There are alternative approaches to most things and there are wonderful supplements for preventing prostate cancer and possibly treating it. I will address this in the chapter on the andropause. I will also repeat my concerns about the actual cause of prostate cancer, since it is such an important issue.

CHAPTER 11

SUSAN B. and POST-PARTUM DEPRESSION

When I first started to write this book, the headlines were filled with news of the trial of Andrea Yates, the woman who struggled with post-partum depression and eventually drowned her five children. Although I think Yates' problems went well beyond post-partum depression, it was a major factor in her breakdown. This is a very real condition that causes untold misery to new mothers. Fortunately, it is easy to treat.

Susan B. found a solution to her post-partum depression by balancing her hormones. I hope her experience will be instructive to other mothers, particularly breastfeeding mothers, who can avoid the side effects of psychogenic drugs by taking this approach.

Depression has been a problem in my family for a long time. My mother and sister and I seemed always to be depressed when I was growing up. Eventually my mother committed suicide, when I was 16 years old.

Along with our depression went low metabolism and in my case, I can't remember when I wasn't battling my weight. I ate normal amounts of food but I was always fat.

Once, as an adult, I got so fed up with always being fat that I went on this rigorous program, exercising three hours a day, six days a week. I did slim down, of course. But it was impossible to keep up that kind of schedule. As soon as I slacked off even a little bit, the weight came right back on.

At the age of 45 I had a child. The moment she was born, I went into a massive depression. It was difficult caring for the baby because I didn't feel any of the joy of motherhood, but I still had all of the daily responsibilities. One day I was talking to my doctor about my depression, complaining a bit about how being overweight contributed to my overall feelings of hopelessness. She told me about other patients of hers who had taken off weight by going to Dr. Platt. I decided to go see him, figuring that slimming down would be one way of improving my situation. Little did I realize it would be the solution to my depression, too.

I was a size 20 when I went to see him. I weighed 190 pounds— it was hard just moving around with that much weight on my 5'3" frame. At first I just went on the diet and held off taking the hormones he had recommended. After a few months I lost 22 pounds.

At that point Dr. Platt said I had to start progesterone and thyroid. So he started me on both of those and my God, what a difference it made in my mood! It was an incredible difference. I feel like I'm a different person today, like a person I haven't seen in about 10 years.

Two months after starting the hormones I was able to start weaning off my prescription anti-depressants.

With the progesterone and the thyroid medication, I had lots of energy and a whole new outlook on life. The other beneficial thing was what it did for my skin. My skin looked so much better after I started the progesterone. It became more radiant, which is a great thing to have happen at my age. I used to have all of these skin tags on my neck and about a month after I started the progesterone they all disappeared.

Ultimately, it took me 10 months to lose about 60 pounds and get down to a size 4. I must have gained a lot of muscle mass, because I don't weigh 105 pounds like most size 4 women. I weigh 137 pounds. Of course, with more muscle mass my metabolism is much higher than it used to be, so it's that much easier to maintain my weight while still eating the foods I love to eat.

A LIFETIME BATTLING OBESITY

Susan B. is another example of someone who fought obesity her entire life, not because of an eating problem, but because of a hormone problem.

She had the classic history of someone with a low progesterone level who becomes estrogen-dominant and depressed. I believe the only cause for post-partum depression is low progesterone. As I have said before, in the third trimester of pregnancy the placenta pours out progesterone, which is why women feel so good at this time during their pregnancy. Then, once the baby is delivered, progesterone levels go down.

For most women, once they start ovulating again their bodies begin producing progesterone and their moods lift. But in Susan's case, she was low in progesterone to begin with, and there she was in her 40s, when hormone levels are on the decline anyway. So she had no source of progesterone.

She also had the classic symptoms of an under-active thyroid: dry skin, her nails didn't grow well, she was easily fatigued, and so on. Her blood tests bore out this deficiency. Her low thyroid contributed to her depression, too. The thyroid has a tremendous influence on metabolism in every cell of the body, including all of the brain cells.

Helping Susan was a very simple matter. As soon as her hormones were balanced she regained a zest for living. The weight loss made her feel even better. It was a particularly sweet reward for a woman who had spent half a lifetime struggling with obesity. And again, it was another classic example of a deficiency of hormones creating havoc with one's health.

Her low progesterone created high insulin levels—the number one cause of obesity. Low progesterone also led to an increase in estrogen—another hormone that creates fat. Low progesterone leads to depression and other psychological problems.

She also had a problem with low thyroid, which lowered her metabolism. Not only did this cause problems with her weight, but it also contributed to her depression.

I hope you, the reader, are beginning to understand the importance of hormones when it comes to health. Susan's case is another classic example that illustrates the importance of being proactive with your own health care. For the most part, you can not expect the medical community to come up with the answers that it may be ill-equipped to find.

EVEN MOVIE STARS GET THE BLUES

As many of you are aware, Brooke Shields has written a book detailing her experience with severe post-partum depression. Her advice to the women with this problem is to avail themselves of anti-depressant medications to alleviate the condition. She has been on multiple talk shows reiterating this advice.

What she has done is to provide the classic, standard medical care approach—take a band-aid (drug) for your problem.

It is my understanding that Ms. Shields utilized in vitro fertilization to get pregnant. The number one reason why woman cannot get pregnant is a low progesterone level. I would guess that she had a rough time with morning sickness—again, the only cause for this is a low progesterone level. After her delivery, her progesterone level dropped to nonexistent levels and precipitated her severe post-partum depression.

The utilization of natural, bio-identical progesterone would have eliminated any need for in vitro fertilization, prevented any morning (or evening) sickness and post-partum depression.

In Brooke Shields' case, giving her progesterone would have eliminated her depression almost immediately.

There is sort of an ironic twist to this situation. Many of you might be aware that Tom Cruise, a scientologist, imposed his own advice to Ms. Shields by recommending a more natural approach—healing with prayer, etc.

Interestingly, Tom Cruise admits that he has a problem with ADHD (Attention Deficit Hyperactivity Disorder). So now you have Brooke Shields with a condition solely caused by a low progesterone level, and Tom Cruise with ADHD—a condition I feel is also caused by a low progesterone level. They both have the same hormone deficiency, yet neither one of them is aware of it, and they both have access to the best medical advice in the world.

Leaves little chance of hope for most people. However, your chances of getting healthy will, in all likelihood, be much better than Ms. Shields or Mr. Cruise. If Ms. Shields had utilized natural progesterone, she might have utilized the same title for her book as I have.

CHAPTER 12

ATTENTION DEFICIT DISORDER (ADD) and ATTENTION DEFICIT HYPERACTIVITY DISORDER (ADHD)

THE SILENT EPIDEMIC

I could not write a book about the influence of hormones without making special mention of attention deficit disorder (ADD) and attention deficit hyperactivity disorder (ADHD).

These are two conditions that I feel are primarily related to hormonal imbalance.

There are many kids struggling in school today because of difficulties focusing. Often, the reason for this inability to pay attention in class or to do homework is that they might be hypoglycemic. Any time sugar is taken from the brain, it cannot focus. The reason for the low sugars is that they are over-producing insulin. Because of hypoglycemia there is a persistent craving for foods that provide sugar i.e. fruit juice, soda, candy, etc.

Very often kids with ADD have a weight problem since they are continuously eating high glycemic carbohydrates.

So what about ADHD? This condition starts out the same way—too much insulin leading to low sugar levels. However, kids with ADHD have to contend with another hormone: adrenalin.

The brain cannot function without sugar. The body has an amazing capacity for raising sugar levels. Prominent among these regulatory reactions is a process called gluconeogenesis. Simply put, this is the process of creating sugar from protein. It is mediated through the sympathetic nervous system. In other words, the body pours out adrenalin to raise sugar levels. Adrenalin, which is natural speed, causes these kids to be hyperactive.

At the same time the body is creating adrenalin, the low sugar levels create cravings for food high in sugar. Ingestion of sugar then leads to the over-production of insulin, leading to a drop in sugar, leading to difficulty focusing, leading to the over-production of adrenalin, leading to hyperactive behavior and on and on.

Kids with ADHD are usually thin. The hyperactivity burns up the sugar before it's converted to fat for storage. Often times the hyperactivity is masked by the child being actively involved in sports.

Kids with ADHD are treated with drugs such as Ritalin, Adderal, Strattera, etc. However, approaching these conditions from a hormonal standpoint eliminates these conditions in most cases without having to resort to medication.

If you have been paying attention to prior chapters, the missing hormone that causes ADD and ADHD should be known to you—namely, progesterone. Hormones are inherited from either parent. If a mother is estrogen dominant, i.e. painful periods, breast tenderness, PMS, morning sickness with pregnancies, etc, she is low in progesterone. This can be passed on to her daughter or son. Again, anyone with a low progesterone level will over-produce insulin, thereby causing hypoglycemia, leading to ADD.

There are many adults with undiagnosed ADD or ADHD. People who experience sleepiness between 3 and 4 in the afternoon or while driving—this is ADD. Very often, people who become workaholics may actually have ADHD and are living on high levels of adrenalin caused by recurrent hypoglycemia.

I had an experience with a male patient who was about 53. After starting on progesterone his immediate response was that it made him extremely tired. As soon as he said that I realized he was an adult ADHD. He was a trim male, working a 12-14 hour day. When I placed him on progesterone this prevented his insulin levels from rising. It took away his hypoglycemia and so his adrenalin levels went down. This was a man who lived on high adrenalin levels all his life. All of a sudden he got exposed to the lower levels of adrenalin that you and I are used to—but he wasn't.

I predict that 30 years from now someone will get the Nobel Prize for figuring out the cause of ADD and ADHD. It may take that long before doctors realize that children have hormones, just like adults.

In the meantime, it would be helpful if schools eliminated

vending machines with sodas, juice, candy, chips, etc., which are exacerbating the problem. Classes focusing on nutrition would provide a lifelong benefit to children.

ADHD IN ADULTS

I debated a long time about whether to include ADD and ADHD in this book. If one was to ask specialists in this field what causes this problem they will admit that they do not know. As far as I know, I am the only doctor in the world that approaches this from a hormonal standpoint. Simply put, too little progesterone, too much insulin and too much adrenalin. My philosophy is so far removed from the standard of medical practice, which calls for the use of dangerous stimulants to treat this, that it can create concerns for traditional practitioners. However, my goal is not to assuage the ego of doctors, it is to get my patients better by treating the cause of illness.

I do not treat small children that are hyperactive in my practice—but I do treat their parents. If there is a hyperactive child at home then one, or both, of the parents is also ADHD. If the child is adopted, then he or she almost has a 100% chance of being ADHD because most (not all) people who give up their children for adoption are young mothers who have gotten into drugs and alcohol and got pregnant. Most children who get involved with drugs and alcohol are ADHD. Later on I plan to devote an entire book to ADD/ADHD and will explain my clinical observations more in depth.

It is reasonable to assume that children with ADHD grow up to be adults with ADHD. It should not be surprising to note that most adults with ADHD are un-recognized by the medical community. It should not be surprising that many conditions associated with adult ADHD are considered incurable by the medical community because we are dealing with hormones out of balance; an uncomfortable concept for many physicians.

The typical adult with ADHD will have a history of increased physical activity as a teenager being slim during his or her youth, never opening a book in high school or college until the night before an exam, may possibly have become a type A personality or workaholic. There will be a history of being easily irritated, quick to anger, possibly road rage; they might have high expectations of other people. As they approach their middle years they start putting on weight around the middle. They will have symptoms of hypoglycemia with sleepiness in the late afternoon, or while driving, or after eating.

They commonly display restless activity—tapping their fingers, moving their foot while sitting, and at times have symptoms of restless leg syndrome at night or just plain restlessness.

Commonly associated conditions are type II diabetes and also fibromyalgia. Many patients I see in my practice are unrecognized adults with ADHD, which means there is a strong family history of associated hormonal problems—a mother with breast cancer, a sister with endometriosis, a brother with bipolar disorder, and, certainly, their children or nephews and nieces who are hyperactive (ADHD).

All the conditions associated with ADHD are considered for the most part incurable—ADHD itself, restless leg syndrome, fibromyalgia, type II diabetes, endometriosis, menstrual migraines, asthma, etc. And yet, utilizing natural bio-identical hormones, altering a patient's eating habits, and providing insight, often lead to a 'miraculous' resolution of these problems.

In the future, for those who might be interested, I will go

into an in depth approach and analysis of this topic. My goal
for the present book is to introduce to people the idea of utilizing natural hormones for wellness.

CHAPTER 13

HORMONAL IMBALANCES IN CHILDREN

We are about to enter uncharted territory, because the relationship of childhood illness and hormonal influence has essentially been ignored. What I will be stating here is based primarily on logic and my own clinical observations; there are no studies to fall back on.

What I will be discussing are my own personal observations.

Before we start, I want to remind the reader of a number of truisms:

1.   Hormones control every system of the body

2. Males and females have the same hormones but have different levels

3. Hormones are inherited from either parent

4. At different stages in life, hormone levels vary

This book is not intended to be a textbook of medicine. And in no way is it offered to replace discussions with your family doctor. My goal is to provide the reader with insight into the mechanics of the body, so they can have a better understanding of why they or their child may be having problems.

Just as with adults, an imbalance of one hormone in children often leads to an imbalance of other hormones as the body tries to adjust to a deficiency.

Most people are aware that we have a nationwide problem with overweight or obese children. Along with these statistics we are beginning to see a significant increase in attention deficit disorder. Female children who have started their periods may be experiencing irregular menses, severe cramps, migraines, or other symptoms. This chapter will address these problems.

THE MISSING LINK

It is apparent to me that an over-production of a single hormone is associated with creating many metabolic problems. This hormone is insulin. Insulin is the number one hormone that creates fat, especially around the middle. It is the number one hormone that creates type II diabetes, and it is the hormone that creates ADD and ADHD. There is a separate chapter devoted to this problem in which I explain the hormonal difference between ADD and ADHD.

If one is willing to accept that too much insulin is creating problems, then let's go one step further. Why is the body over-producing insulin? Although the over-production of insulin in children is multi-factorial, it can probably be blamed on two main influences. The first, and not necessarily the most important, is the type of food children get exposed to. Too many carbohydrates in the form of fruit juice, soda, chips, fries, candy, cookies, etc., leading to high sugar levels and subsequently, over-production of insulin which then puts the sugar into the fat cells.

The other factor, which may be the proximal cause for these problems, is a deficiency of progesterone in these children. I consider this the missing link.

A deficiency of progesterone is almost always associated with an over-production of insulin. If a mother (or father) is low in progesterone, they can pass this trait onto their child. A mother low in progesterone would have a history of estrogen domi-nance—cramps, PMS, breast tenderness, nausea with pregnancy, fibroids, fibrocystic disease, migraine headaches, etc.

My own mother was estrogen-dominant and wound up dying of breast cancer because of it. She had thin arms and legs and a large abdomen—classic for hyperinsulinemia secondary to low progesterone. I inherited a progesterone deficiency from her. I had ADD as a child—I used to get up and walk out of class and could not focus. They didn't diagnose ADD back then; they thought I was bored. I wasn't bored—I just couldn't pay attention. I was continuously hypoglycemic—I craved sweets. I used to steal candy from candy stores (I hope Mr. Birnbaum is not reading this). I rarely studied in high school or college, except the night before exams. I could only focus on things that interested me, like early rock and roll in high school, and bridge and poker in college. Please note: I studied 6 hours every night in medical school—but I was interested in medicine.

I have fought with weight all my life because I have over-produced insulin. When I first went into practice, I used to nod off between 3 and 4p.m.—sometimes while talking to patients! Oftentimes when I was driving I had to slap my face to keep my eyes open. All these symptoms disappeared after I started using natural progesterone.

What I am proposing is that a factor linking many of the problems children experience may possibly be related to a low progesterone production.

THE OVERWEIGHT CHILD

When people are young, it is often possible to get fat to melt off their bodies. They have not yet reached the stage where their bodies become sophisticated, efficient machines for fat-production and maintenance of fat.

The last chapter of this book deals with weight control—the approach to children is similar to adults, but it is easier. Very often, just teaching the child and/or the parents how to eat is all that's required. Instructing them on the importance of exercise—primarily to burn sugar rather than fat—is mandatory. Adjusting hormones such as progesterone and thyroid may be necessary. Eliminating unnecessary medications, where possible, is helpful.

What would be of immeasurable benefit is to get parents united to eliminate the candy-juice-soda machines in the school, and to work with the dietitians in the school and the fast-food purveyors outside the school to offer lower-carb choices.

PUTTING PERIODS IN PERSPECTIVE

If the ovaries are not producing an adequate amount of progesterone, the pituitary sends out hormones to up the production. In many cases the ovaries, for genetic reasons, are not capable of increasing progesterone, but the extra stimulation increases the amount of estrogen. This extra estrogen, without the proper balance of progesterone, can result in estrogen dominance. This condition is associated with a number of symptoms—cramps, PMS, breast tenderness, menstrual headaches, etc. This excess estrogen can wind up creating fat around the hips and buttocks. Low progesterone leading to increased estrogen stimulation can lead to fibroids in the uterus and cysts on the ovaries and in the breast. Cysts in the ovaries can produce an excess of testosterone causing problems with acne and excessive hair growth. They call this polycystic ovarian syndrome (PCOS)—again, most likely caused by a deficiency of progesterone. Keep in mind, the low progesterone associated with all of the above changes is causing more insulin to be produced, creating weight around the middle.

WHAT TO DO

Again, let me remind you that I am providing you with my interpretation of how the body is working and why your child may be having problems.

The concept of treating people—adults and/or children—with bio-identical natural hormones is unknown to most doctors because they were never given the information and knowledge to do so. I was never provided with any information in medical school, medical textbooks, or medical journals about the use of natural hormones.

Do not be concerned if your physician appears resistant to the concept—he or she will eventually accept it because it will become the standard of medical practice. Contact with a compound pharmacy can point you in the direction of a physician who may be more receptive at this time.

Very often teenage girls with menstrual problems are put on birth control pills to help with cramps or acne. This is the classic medical approach to treating people with band-aids instead of dealing with the cause of the problem.

The cause of their problem is a reduced level of progesterone. The only time a female produces progesterone is during ovulation. Birth control pills prevent the ovaries from ovulating—so these girls go from low levels of progesterone to none. Keep in mind, progesterone is one of the most important hormones in the female body.

Giving natural, bio-identical progesterone cream (not over-the-counter, because it is too weak) will eliminate cramps, PMS, migraine headaches, and asthma; it will lower insulin levels and help eliminate fat, ADD and ADHD; it will help clear up acne and improve PCOS. Dosage: Progesterone Cream 100mg (¼ TSP)—apply twice a day to forearm and wrist on days 7 thru 28 of the cycle.

FINAL THOUGHTS

I am very aware that I am touching on controversial areas by making recommendations on treating conditions in children with natural hormones where there have been no studies. People need to realize that the major funding for studies come via drug companies, and it is important that they do their studies. However, they are unable to patent natural products so it is unlikely that we will see studies pertaining to natural hormones in children for a long time. Used correctly, natural progesterone is nontoxic. Fetuses in the womb get exposed to extremely high levels of progesterone, which aids in brain development, etc.

I have recommended natural progesterone in children as young as nine years old—one child had ADD and was failing in school. Several months later he was an 'A' student. Another was a girl nine years old who was having monthly migraine headaches. She had already started developing breasts and was evidently estrogen dominant (like her mother). After starting progesterone, her migraine headaches disappeared.

Children with undiagnosed hormonal problems can look forward to a multitude of lifelong difficulties. Children with ADD can wind up with diabetes, weight problems, and difficulty holding jobs. Children with ADHD often become adults with Type A personalities—workaholics—and may wind up with bipolar disorder. They frequently develop chemical dependency to alcohol, cigarettes, methamphetamine, and other substances.

Girls with low progesterone/high estrogen will have difficulty getting pregnant and will have miscarriages, morning sickness, postpartum depression, fibroids, endometriosis, asthma, migraine headaches, breast cancer, weight problems, and other difficulties.

The fact is that children are being exposed to toxic drugs such as anti-depressants, birth control pills, and stimulants for hyper-activity. Wouldn't it be more beneficial to treat the actual cause of their problems with the identical natural hormone that is missing? Very often hormonal problems lead to depression in children. Children are also prone to thyroid conditions. Covering everything goes way beyond the scope of this book. I am only attempting to introduce the idea that hormonal imbalance may be affecting the health of children. Perhaps children should experience the miracle of bio-identical hormones.

CHAPTER 14

KAREN H. and MIGRAINE HEADACHES

Karen is a fashionable woman in her 50's who came to me to solve a post-menopausal weight problem. Her medical history indicated that she'd suffered from migraine headaches all her life. She was amazed when I told her that the migraines were curable. She'd tried to get help with them, spending a considerable amount of money, but to no avail. Readers who have been tolerating migraines should learn from her example: it's never too late to defeat an old enemy like migraines, although the earlier you address this problem the better.

I've gotten migraine headaches about three or four times a month for my entire life. There would be this intense throbbing behind my right eyeball, in my temples, a neck ache and nausea. Doctors didn't diagnose these headaches as migraines because I didn't see "auras"— the white light migraine sufferers typically see. I also was not sensitive to light and I did not need to go into a dark room. But later, in my fifties, a neurosurgeon told me they were migraines.

So when I was young I just called them "my headaches" and took codeine to lessen the pain. When I was 29 years old, I had one so bad that it sent me to the emergency room at the local hospital. I was vomiting, the pain was excruciating and I thought, 'Nobody has headaches like this. "I asked my friend to drive me to the emergency room. They treated me with a muscle relaxant and Valium. The next day I just soldiered on and went to work.

The second time I went to the emergency room with a migraine, one of the doctors said it was a severe sinus headache and he recommended nose surgery. I did have nose surgery and it didn't do a thing.

The third time a migraine sent me to the hospital, the doctors wouldn't let me leave without doing a spinal tap on me. My symptoms were nearly identical to what you see in people who are about to have a stroke, an aneurysm, or who have spinal meningitis. That gives you an idea of how severe the migraines were.

I was told the headaches might go away after menopause, but they didn't. When menopause failed to give me relief I finally went to see a neurosurgeon. My headaches were diagnosed as migraines and I was given two medications that finally helped. He gave me Inderal and Imitrex. The Inderal reduced the frequency of the headaches to once every six weeks or so, which was a blessing. Whenever I did feel a headache coming on, I would self-inject the Imitrex, which would stop the progression and leave me without pain.

Naturally, I was grateful for this relief after all those years of suffering. But I would later find out that Inderal and Imitrex were just masking the pain, not getting to the cause of it.

Meanwhile, I stopped smoking. The combination of stopping smoking and going through menopause caused me to gain 50 pounds. This was scary to me. I had always been pretty close to the weight I wanted to be. I was one of those Twiggy generation people who was always trying to lose 10 pounds—you can never be quite thin enough, but generally speaking I didn't have a weight problem. But once I had gained the 50 pounds I was scared. I looked matronly, felt old and I didn't know whether I would ever be able to lose this weight.

I heard a friend talking about Dr. Platt and she spoke so highly of him that I decided to go to him for weight loss.

I went to see him and we talked for an hour. I was comfortable with him and I was fascinated that he's a traditionally trained M.D. who has a philosophy that crosses over into alternative medicine. He told me he could eliminate my migraine headaches and that losing the 50 pounds would just be the icing on the cake.

He put me on progesterone, thyroid medication and DHEA and started weaning me off the Inderal as well as the HRT my gynecologist had put me on at menopause.

At some point during the weaning from Inderal I had a terrible, terrible night when I couldn't put my head on a pillow because my head hurt so much. It wasn't like a migraine; it was like every one of my hairs hurt my scalp. If I touched my hair, my scalp was in agony. I spent the night sitting up, catching whatever sleep I could, and the next morning I called Dr. Platt's office and went to see him.

He told me that what was happening was that I was getting my nerve endings back. The drugs I'd been taking had numbed them and now they were coming back to life. He told me the symptoms would be gone within 36 hours and he was right. It is now 20 months since I first saw Dr. Platt and I have not had a single migraine headache.

It was also the easiest weight loss I have ever experienced. I stuck to the diet religiously and the pounds just melted off. I lost eight pounds the first week and about three pounds every successive week. I started in

September and by Thanksgiving I'd lost 32 pounds. I felt great, I was-
n't hungry, and I wasn't getting headaches! At Thanksgiving I went
off the diet because I had tons of guests and relatives coming in for the
holidays, and my passion is cooking for people. But I plan to go back
on the diet at some point to lose the last 18 pounds.

The weight I lost was a different kind of 32 pounds—I can't
quite explain it but I had this feeling that I was losing stored-up fat
from a long time ago. There was a different definition to my body. It
looked and felt different.

The other day I was cleaning out my medicine cabinet and I came
upon some Imitrex shots that were still good. One part of me wanted to
keep them—what if I got another headache? These things were life-
savers at one point in my life. But I had the courage to throw them out.
I've been headache-free for 20 months, through all kinds of changes in
my diet, and I don't see any reason why that should change.

PROGESTERONE AND MIGRAINES

Karen is another example of a woman who had been estrogen-
dominant her entire life. Estrogen is very damaging to blood
vessels and migraine headaches are another result of the adverse
effect of estrogen on blood vessels.

You might ask, why did Karen feel the toxicity of estrogen as
migraines, while someone like Brenda J. experienced it in the
form of fibroid tumors and troubled pregnancies? As I've
explained before, there are receptor sites for hormones all over the
body and people vary regarding where they have receptor sites.
Likewise, symptoms will vary according to where particular sites
are located. I suppose one could say that Karen was lucky her
excess estrogen didn't eventually cause her to have breast or ovarian cancer. However, you'd have had a hard time convincing
Karen of her good luck in the middle of a migraine attack. Those
are brutal. I once treated a woman who had severe menstrual

migraines starting at age 14 with her first menses. On two occasions she had paralytic migraines resulting in strokes.

Everyone knows somebody who has migraines. And everyone knows how excruciating they are, so it's quite remarkable that the medical community has missed the simple fact that natural progesterone is a cost-effective cure for menstrual migraines. Most doctors simply don't know enough about hormones to help all the millions of women out there like Karen. These women are desperate for relief. Many of them attend "pain clinics" and explore every avenue they can—meditation, acupressure and so on—but continue to suffer month after month.

Karen went all the way from her teenage years—when her body *first* started producing estrogen—to menopause suffering from these headaches. At menopause, she would have had hope of getting some relief, now that her body was reducing its production of estrogen, but doctors placed her on HRT and made sure the migraines continued.

All she needed to solve a lifelong problem was progesterone. This is the hormone that protects women from the effects of too much estrogen. As long as she continues taking it, Karen won't have any more migraine headaches.

She also had a low thyroid, which isn't surprising in someone with low progesterone levels, because progesterone has a major influence on the thyroid. Giving her the right thyroid medication helped her to lose weight in a comfortable fashion.

When Karen talks about feeling as though she was losing stored-up fat and seeing her body change in a way she had not seen before, she is just talking about the difference between a fat-burning weight loss program and a muscle-burning calorie restriction diet. In her youth, Karen did a lot of calorie restriction diets—those grapefruit-and-lean-meat diets that were popular in the 1960s and 1970s. Those make you lose muscle. They give you a sagging look, make your skin look droopy and impair muscle tone. To Karen, actually losing fat and seeing some muscle definition was a revelation.

Would it be fair to say that Karen felt eliminating her migraine headaches with a natural, bio-identical hormone was a miracle?

CHAPTER 15

WHY WE DON'T HAVE PREVENTIVE MEDICINE IN THIS COUNTRY

One can say that there is almost no such thing as preventive medicine in this country. When you talk to most doctors about preventive medicine they think you're talking about giving flu shots. However, most people believe that preventive medicine is preventing heart attacks, strokes, cancer, diabetes, etc.

If we look at statistics, it becomes clear that over the past 60 years there's been hardly any diminution in the incidence of any of these conditions. Despite the proliferation of drugs and new medical technology, nothing much has changed.

NO PROFIT MOTIVE

Almost everything doctors learn in medical school about treating patients is based on research done by drug companies. This is why most doctors have little basic knowledge of natural hormones—drug companies cannot patent natural products. Even endocrinologists, who specialize in hormones, for the most part only feel comfortable using the synthetic hormones produced by drug companies, not the natural hormones produced by the body.

Along these same lines, doctors learn little preventive medicine in medical school because drug companies have no interest in preventing disease—why should they? There's no profit for drug companies in treating the root causes of heart attacks, strokes, diabetes and cancer. The entire medical establishment is geared toward treatment, not prevention. For the most part, drug companies develop drugs to treat symptoms of disease. Antibiotics are the only drugs that cure disease.

Even insurance companies—which have the most to gain from doctors practicing effective preventive medicine—play into this system by discounting the importance of proper screening procedures. By and large, insurance companies are loath to pay for simple screening tests. These are the kinds of tests that could help patients head off diseases they might be prone to developing. When a doctor or patient requests coverage for a blood test or any other study, the insurance company normally responds by asking for a diagnosis to support the doctor's reason for doing the test.

Well, if you had the diagnosis, the patient would already have the disease. The whole point of screening is to prevent the disease from coming on in the first place.

There is a blood test called a CA-125 that allows doctors to screen for cancer of the ovaries. Cancer of the ovaries is a condition that is 100% curable if it's found early and almost

100% fatal after it's spread. Insurance companies will not cover a CA-*125* as a screening test but will pay for it once you have the condition.

This is especially galling in light of how eager the medical community is to place women on estrogen, a substance that places them at serious risk for cancer of the ovaries. Estrogen is still one of the largest selling drugs in the world. You would think a simple, inexpensive test for cancer of the ovaries would be standard in a society that prescribes estrogen with such regularity. However, for reasons I cannot decipher, insurance companies will pay for PSA tests to screen for prostate cancer, but not for a CA-125 test.

STROKES AND HEART DISEASE

Heart attacks are the number one cause of death, both in men and women. This would, of course, be a prime area to incorporate the concept of preventive medicine. And yet, in spite of all the measures being implemented—coronary bypass surgery, the placing of stents, angioplasty, the use of drugs to lower cholesterol, stop smoking campaigns, dieting and exercise programs, etc.—there has been no change in the cardiovascular mortality rate since 1950.

Is it possible that we are not addressing the major causes of cardiovascular disease?

Everybody has heard about cholesterol—the good (HDL) and the bad (LDL), etc. Lipitor is now the largest selling drug in the world. This factor has been greatly enhanced by the tendency to keep on lowering the upper limits of normal in terms of total cholesterol. When I was in medical school normal cholesterol levels went up to 300. This level has been continuously lowered to the latest "normal" level of 180.

Interestingly, they have never been able to demonstrate

convincingly that lowering cholesterol prevents coronary artery disease and some studies indicate that more people have heart attacks with low cholesterol than high cholesterol. There is, however, a much more serious risk factor that has been largely ignored by the medical community—the homocysteine level.

Homocysteine is found in everybody's bloodstream. It is a breakdown product of methionine, an amino acid. In high levels it creates damage to blood vessels and causes them to be sticky—a risk factor for cholesterol plaques and blood clots. It predisposes not only to heart attacks, but to strokes, Alzheimer's disease, Parkinson's disease, osteoporosis, and it shortens the lifespan. Certainly, its its an important risk factor to screen for, but there's a problem. The treatment consists of a combination of three B vitamins—folic acid, vitamin B12 and vitamin B6, along with trimethylglycine—natural products of little benefit to drug companies.

The usual scenario seems to be if there is no interest by drug companies, doctors rarely are aware of the problem. Even if they are aware, insurance companies do not pay for this test unless there is an underlying diagnosis to support doing the test.

There is another risk factor that is often not considered, called C-reactive protein (C-RP). This is a marker for inflammation in the coronary arteries; again, a situation predisposing to plaque formation and blood clots. Women with elevated C-RP levels are at significant risk of sudden death and this element is considered a much greater risk factor than LDL cholesterol.

As an aside, elevations of C-RP can also be a marker for cancer of the colon and macular degeneration, the number one cause of adult-onset blindness. Certainly, this is a screening test that should be performed, but is rarely done so. The treatment of elevated levels often incorporates the use of natural antioxidants, which are again substances that are not promoted by pharmaceutical companies.

THE MESSAGE

People have to understand that many times, in order to be healthy, they have to become pro-active. They have to take their health into their own hands. They cannot fully rely on a health system that is not fully committed to their being healthy.

Eventually, doctors will be tuned into the use of natural hormones to prevent and heal illnesses and to screen for other preventable disorders. However, this will not happen until patients demand a better approach to their health.

CHAPTER 16

JANET L. and FIBROMYALGIA

Fibromyalgia is rheumatism of the muscles, ligaments and tendons. It is far more common than most people realize. It can cause crippling pain that makes normal activity excruciating. I see many patients with this malady. It seems to occur with great frequency among overweight people. It can be healed using a natural, drugless approach, a fact that should bring joy to the hearts of many sufferers. I hope Janet's story will inspire others to say "no" to this debilitating condition and release themselves into a pain-free, joyous life.

I've had fibromyalgia for 20 years, although it wasn't diagnosed until recently. Most people who have fibromyalgia do not get properly diagnosed until they have had it for at least seven years. That's because

*it is a progressive disease and when it starts out it might only mani-
fest as a stiff neck or isolated pain and general fatigue. The symptoms,
in other words, are so general they can be interpreted as the flu, tired
muscles, a sleep disorder or any number of less serious problems.*

*When I first started experiencing the pain of fibromyalgia I was
living in the mountains in Washington State. In that often cold, usually moist climate my body behaved like a barometer—whenever the
weather changed my body would feel it. Whether it was dampness,
cold, a change in the wind—any change would register in my body as
pain. I went to rheumatologists, chiropractors, all kinds of doctors
about my pain, but none of them had a solution for me.*

*One doctor started me on cortisone shots. We reached a point where
he was shooting cortisone into 42 muscles in my back every day. He
finally said, "Janet, I can't do this any more. You've become a human
pincushion."*

*I would have good days and bad days. On my good days I was
energetic and took part in family activities with great zest. On bad
days I wouldn't be able to get dressed without stopping a few times to
lie down and rest and get my energy back.*

*In the days before the fibromyalgia was advanced, my husband and
I decided to build our dream house up in the mountains in Cardiff. I took
a very active part in designing it, a house on three levels. It was a proj-
ect that went on for several years. By the time we were close to finishing
it, the major symptoms of my fibromyalgia had set in. At that point, I
found it unbearable to climb stairs. I had to wonder who that person was
who had thought to design a three-story house. But no one had diagnosed
me or told me my problem would get worse every year.*

*I was given various medications for pain, Neurontin being the one
I ended up taking long-term. It dulled the pain without getting at the
source of the problem.*

*The way I dealt with the pain in the early days was to be very
active. Inactivity seemed to exacerbate the stiffness and pain, so I threw
myself into family activities. We have a large extended family up north*

and I loved making dinners and entertaining. I could forget about my pain if I had a goal like cooking for 40 people. However, the activity took a lot out of me and after these dinners were over I would have to recuperate for a week.

Part of the fibromyalgia was a sleeping problem—the pain kept me awake. Often I would get only three hours of sleep at night. I would toss and turn and then finally go to my husband's recliner to get some sleep. It was easier to find a comfortable position. I also started getting migraine headaches.

Gradually I reached the point where I was quite debilitated. If it were snowing outside I could only walk a half a block or so before exhaustion would set in. My knees would get so swollen they were like footballs. I couldn't bend them.

A rheumatologist finally diagnosed me. He checked my pressure points and told me all 18 of them were inflamed. He said I had both osteoarthritis and fibromyalgia.

I finally had a diagnosis, but the rheumatologist didn't have a solution for my pain. He just prescribed more Neurontin. My husband and I arrived at the point where we were ready to sacrifice our dream house so we could live in a warm, dry climate where I could be in less pain. We sold our house in Cardiff and bought a house in the desert. As soon as we'd moved in I contacted a rheumatologist—I needed a local source for my Neurontin. This doctor checked my pressure points and they were, as usual, inflamed.

Meanwhile, I happened to see Dr. Platt on television talking about hormones and weight loss. I thought that if I could lose some weight I might be able to move around better. I weighed 185 back then and I am 5 feet tall. The weight seemed to exacerbate my pain. So I decided to go in to see him.

He was astounding. I sat and talked to him for <u>two and a half hours for my first visit</u>! He went over all my records and then he started asking me such pointed questions that I kept on saying to myself "How did he know that?"

He told me I was internalizing anger and that I needed to face what was angering me and to cope with it. We talked about some fairly personal stuff. He gave me some ideas for changing patterns in my life that were forcing me to swallow all this anger. He said that I could put the fibromyalgia into remission through lifestyles changes and balancing my hormones.

I started taking progesterone and I went on the diet. Three weeks after seeing Dr. Platt I went to see the rheumatologist. He checked my pressure points and told me there was no more inflammation. I told him that for the first time I was able to sleep through the night and that I didn't have pain any more. This was three weeks after starting the progesterone! The rheumatologist said "Whatever you're doing, continue doing it. Your osteoarthritis has gone into remission."

I got really excited about how effective the progesterone had been. The next time I went in to see Dr. Platt I wanted to have a whole blood panel done. If one hormone could take away all that pain, what else could we accomplish by balancing all of my hormones?

When he examined my blood panel, Dr. Platt said that I had a thyroid deficiency. He gave me a prescription for thyroid medication and my energy level increased dramatically. I continued with the diet, eventually losing 53 pounds. Today I weigh 132 and I feel so incredible, it's as though someone gave me back my life from years ago. I feel young inside. When I visited my grandchildren up north last time I went hiking and swimming with them, things I'd never been able to do. "It's like we have a new grandma!" all the kids said.

Dr. Platt also prescribed testosterone, which has given me back my sex life—my husband is absolutely thrilled.

I feel so blessed to have met Dr. Platt. He's changed my life. Some of my friends ask me whether I'd have sold my dream house it I'd known I was going to feel this good—today I'd have no problem with those three flights of stairs. But I know everything happens for a reason. I'm just grateful things have turned out the way they have.

AN UNDER-RECOGNIZED DISEASE

Janet's long and unsuccessful quest to get help with her fibromyalgia doesn't surprise me at all. Only about 50 percent of doctors even acknowledge the reality of fibromyalgia. Even if they make the diagnosis, they will then tell their patients that there's no known cure for it. The reason that they cannot cure it is because doctors do not understand the cause of it. If you don't understand what causes something, how can you get rid of it?

Of course there's a cause for it. In my experience a large part of it is caused by internalization of anger. Every patient I've ever treated for fibromyalgia has been a person who internalizes anger.

The classic profile of persons with fibromyalgia is as follows: They are perfectionists who, unfortunately, live in an imperfect world. As perfectionists, they have high expectations of themselves, and of the people living around them. However, they are surrounded by people who are 'flaky,' who have no work ethic, or who are sociopathic and pathological liars. This is what America seems to be made up of nowadays. These kinds of people can never achieve the level of expectations required by perfectionists.

Very often people become perfectionists because they never got enough approval from one or both parents. They were the "good little girls or boys" when they were growing up and continued to be the good little girls or boys as adults. They find it difficult to say no to anyone, always seeking approval. They avoid hassles and confrontations; they become people-pleasers and caregivers to relatives who are sick. The latter causes an exceptionally high level of suppressed anger.

The lack of confrontation and avoidance of hassle causes them to stay in marriages with partners who are wrong for them. News events reinforce the existence of imperfection in the world. An extremely common reason for people to be angry is their weight: every time they look in the mirror or try on clothing, they get angry.

Another common source of fibromyalgia is living with a person who is very controlling. The "victim" is forced to "walk on egg-shells" to avoid displeasing the partner.

The bottom line of fibromyalgia is a loss of control: These are people who allow the rest of the world to control the way they feel, whether that means people who fail to live up to their expectations or unhappiness about their weight, their spouse, their mother (very common), etc. Visualize people with "road rage" who allow other drivers to control how they feel. Instead of "road rage," those people have "life-in-general" rage.

The response to this anger—which often they do not realize they are experiencing because it is internalized—is the general tensing of muscles. When muscles are tensed, two things happen: lactic acid builds up, causing pain (athletes call it muscle burn), and a large amount of energy is expended, causing persistent fatigue.

At night their mind continues to deal with something that is frustrating them or angering them, so all night long their muscles tense. The jaws tighten, causing them to grind their teeth or develop TMJ (temporomandibular joint dysfunction). A lot of anger is internalized into the GI tract, causing problems with constipation and diarrhea, often referred to as IBS (irritable bowel syndrome). People with fibromyalgia awaken during the night with aches and pains: upper back pain, neck pain, low back pain with pain along the side of the hips, etc.

Here you have people who can't say no—the givers—surrounded by takers. They wind up having unwanted house guests, having Thanksgiving and Christmas dinners at their house every year (talk about stress!), taking care of an aging parent, etc.

The epitome of loss of control is living with a controlling

mate. Their victims continually walk around on eggshells with perpetually tensed muscles, whether they are aware of it or not, always trying to please their mate.

And again, perhaps one of the most common examples of loss of control causing anger is the patient who can't lose weight. Here they are, dieting, exercising, cutting out fat, doing everything they think is right, and they cannot lose an ounce. Imagine their anger when they look in the mirror every day. Their inability to lose weight is controlling them.

What I do with these patients is to give them insight into their anger. And I encourage them to find any outlet they can for it, whether it's exercise, whacking a plastic bat against a foam rubber doll, kick-boxing, going to the shooting range, or whatever. I urge them to make changes in their lives—with the help of a therapist, if necessary—to deal with the source of their anger. If they don't deal with the source of their anger, they're going to have fibromyalgia forever. They are instructed to lower their expectations and to remove everybody in their lives that gives them negative energy, or to quit responding to those people. I explain to my patients that I can get hormones into balance, but cannot eliminate anger from their lives. I give them insight on dealing with the sources of their negative energy.

Janet L. and I had discussions about her anger, and she started taking steps to change certain parts of her life. Meanwhile, I explained to her that her under-active thyroid was contributing to her problem. The thyroid gland has a tremendous influence on muscle tissue, and when you're dealing with fibromyalgia, you're dealing with muscle tissue. The condition that creates the greatest muscle damage—more than heart attacks, more than anything else—is an under active thyroid. Every patient I've ever treated for fibromyalgia has had an under-active thyroid.

I put Janet on thyroid medication, and that was the beginning of a healing process for her muscles that eventually left her pain-free. I also prescribed progesterone for her. It's a feel-good hormone that is effective for everyone, especially women.

Janet had a nice response to the hormones, the weight loss, and most especially to getting rid of her anger. Today she's a very happy woman.

CHAPTER 17

THOUGHTS ON CHOLESTEROL

Elevated cholesterol is often a barometer pointing to some underlying problem in the body's metabolic system. It's an extremely complex issue that goes way beyond my goals for this book.

However, I would like to address certain factors.

The liver is the main source of cholesterol and the raw material for making cholesterol is the fat that is stored there. The primary source of this fat is excess carbohydrates that are ingested rather than ingested fat. A study was done at Johns Hopkins University to determine the effect on cholesterol from eating white meat (fish and chicken) versus red meat (all other meats). The result of the study showed that white meat and red meat both *lowered* cholesterol by the same amount.

To a large extent the thyroid gland controls cholesterol metabolism. In fact, I remember when I went to medical school they often referred to cholesterol as "the poor man's thyroid test." Unfortunately, many doctors fail to assess thyroid function when dealing with elevated cholesterol because the emphasis in medicine is to treat the symptom and not the cause. Giving thyroid hormone can very often lower cholesterol levels.

It is estimated that 20 percent of the American population has Syndrome X, a disease of hyperinsulinemia. Insulin puts sugar not only into fat cells, where it gets converted into fat, but also into the liver, where it also is converted into fat. This is the primary fuel for cholesterol. If someone has high cholesterol and also has a low HDL cholesterol and an elevated triglyceride level (the hallmarks of Syndrome X), the lowering of insulin levels often helps in decreasing the cholesterol level.

As people get older, hormone levels go down. Most hormones are made with cholesterol. It has been theorized that part of the reason cholesterol levels rise as we get older is that it is a response by the body to a lowering of our hormones (i.e., to provide more substrate to raise our hormones.) Along these lines, one might anticipate that the replacement of natural hormones might lead to a lowering of cholesterol.

As stated previously, the largest selling drug in the world is Lipitor. Other statin-type drugs for lowering cholesterol include Zocor, Pravachol, Mevacor, Lescol, Crestor, and Vytorin. All these drugs have the same side effects. Keep in mind that most of brain tissue is made up of cholesterol and there are special cells in the brain that produce cholesterol. It is not surprising that taking drugs that prevent cholesterol production can cause brain damage and memory loss. They can also cause damage to the liver, nerves, muscles, and the heart. Severe enough muscle damage can even cause irreversible kidney failure.

Most people are aware of HDL and LDL. These are actually lipoproteins that transport cholesterol throughout the body. Both are necessary for proper health. LDL has the reputation for being "bad" because it can oxidize and cause damage to the coronary arteries. HDL is considered "good" because it prevents LDL from oxidizing: the higher the HDL level, the better. There are studies indicating that more people with low cholesterol levels have heart attacks than those with high levels. If this is the case, then one can surmise that it is not necessarily the level of cholesterol that is present, but whether or not it is being oxidized.

One of the most powerful antioxidants for the heart is Coenzyme Q-10. As people get older, the body produces a decreasing amount of this element.

Statin-drugs lower coenzyme Q10 levels. This produces the majority of the side effects of the medications. Obviously, if you are taking one of these drugs, I would recommend taking coenzyme Q10. It is available in drug stores and health food stores.

Perhaps the utilization of antioxidants by themselves might be of more benefit than lowering cholesterol.

A FRIENDLY WARNING

Many people are aware of Vioxx, a pain medication removed from the market because of cardiac concerns. Recently a jury awarded $253,000,000 to the wife of a patient who had died of a heart attack while on Vioxx. This sum was primarily punitive damages because evidence at the trial indicated that the manufacturer was aware of cardiac problems associated with Vioxx. In point of fact, this was not secret information. The association of Vioxx and heart attacks was generally well publicized but unfortunately not noted by the physicians who prescribed

2.3 billion dollars worth per year. The way I would interpret this situation is that the jury is saying we understand that drugs can cause serious side effects. But they expect that if a drug company knows that a certain segment of a population (e.g. heart patients) should not take a certain drug, then the company should let the FDA and doctors and the drug-taking population know it, too.

That brings us to the medication Zocor, made by the same pharmaceutical company. It is the 2nd largest selling drug after Lipitor, the top seller. Side effects of the drug include brain damage, memory loss, nerve damage, irreversible kidney damage secondary to severe muscle damage, heart damage and sudden death. Most, if not all, of these side effects are related to the lowering of coenzyme Q10—an extremely potent antioxidant that the heart cannot function without. Thirteen years ago the company who manufacturers Zocor received a patent for a new formulation of Zocor that included coenzyme Q10. When the time comes that statin-type drugs start being scrutinized more for safety, this may come back to haunt the manufacturers. It may represent another example of prior knowledge of potential problems, and not publicizing the fact that all people taking statin drugs should probably also be taking coenzyme Q10.

CHAPTER 18

SHIRLEY M.—DOCTORS DON'T ALWAYS LISTEN

Before she came to see me at age 50, Shirley had suffered from asthma and severe headaches for her entire adult life. Doctors were unable to help her with either problem or with the weight gain that started in her 20s.

As I helped Shirley master her weight I was able to remove the cause of her asthma and headaches, too. I only wish she had come to me earlier. She would have been spared a hysterectomy and the removal of her gall bladder. Medical studies have shown that 90% of hysterectomies are not necessary.

Shirley's story should strike a familiar note with patients who, when seeking help from the conventional medical community, feel they are being ignored and misunderstood.

For the first 21 years of my life I was healthy and skinny as a rail. I weighed around 103 pounds. Although I developed asthma as a teenager, other than that, I didn't have a lot of medical problems.

All of that changed after I had my first baby. That's when my weight began to fluctuate and I started experiencing painful headaches. I went from a size three to a 13, and the headaches began affecting my ability to function. After my second pregnancy I went up to a size 18 and the headaches got even worse. I tried living on aspirin to control the pain, but it didn't work.

At the age of 45 I hit a wall with my weight. I'd always followed the Dr. Atkins diet to lose weight, but suddenly it didn't work anymore. So I tried different things. I tried eating small portions, eating low fat, low sugar, whole grains and fresh fruits and vegetables. I tried eating yogurt and popcorn and oatmeal. I thought these foods were good for me and would help me, but all they did was make me bigger.

As I got older my asthma attacks went out of control. It almost seemed as though the more weight I gained, the worse the asthma got. I started carrying my inhaler with me all of the time.

After my third baby I had gained so much weight I lost all the muscle control in my tummy. I was pear-shaped. I had skinny legs, skinny arms and a huge stomach. My doctor at the time told me that if I tried to carry another baby I'd probably drag it on the ground so I decided not to have any more babies. I had my uterus removed. That was in 1988.

I had other medical problems at that time as well. I had to have a bladder operation—it seemed like everything was falling out of me! One day I had an attack, doubling over in pain, a very sharp pain in the whole stomach. I was taken to a doctor who diagnosed gall bladder and scheduled me for surgery. Unfortunately, after that surgery I had constant diarrhea. I also had high cholesterol. All hormones had gone out of whack.

My doctor at the time prescribed Premarin for me and also

Meridia, a diet pill for weight loss (I was up to a size 20). In an attempt to understand my failing health, I was reading a lot and I got hold of some literature that was critical of Premarin. I shared it with this doctor. She told me it was nonsense. She said that since I did not have a uterus I needed estrogen. She changed my Premarin to an estradiol patch, another type of estrogen.

I began waking up every morning with headaches. It got so that I dreaded going to sleep at night because I knew that when I woke up I'd have this excruciating pain. I had no energy and started experiencing hot flashes. When I discussed these symptoms with my doctor and suggested that the estradiol patch and the Meridia might not be helping me, she made me feel like a failure. It was as though it was my fault that I could not lose weight.

I was so worried about my failing health that I started talking to everyone I met looking for advice. Through a compound pharmacist I found my way to Dr. Platt.

At our first meeting, Dr. Platt did a very thorough history on me. He wanted to know everything about my medical history, my parents' medical history, my sister, my husband, everything. He had me take a blood test on my first visit. He did a complete hormone panel and after looking over the results, explained what was going on in my body. He told me that the food I had been eating was affecting my insulin levels. He explained what happens throughout the day when you eat those kinds of foods. He could see from my history and my blood tests that I was already making too much estrogen and certainly didn't need to take more. Dr. Platt was concerned about my daughter as well, since my family has a history of breast cancer and uterine cancer. He told me to stop taking the estradiol and the Meridia and he put both me and my daughter on natural progesterone.

He told me that my other doctor wasn't lying to me; it's just that she was misinformed about natural hormones. He also gave me the book "Metabolic Solutions" that reviewed all the things that he told me *about. He said I was to commit myself to a program that he would design for me. He said I would lose my weight, have more energy, and my headaches and hot flashes would probably go away too.*

A nutritional counselor in his office set a goal weight for me and designed a meal plan that included shopping tips and foods to buy. He told me to wean myself off sugar and caffeine. The day after I saw the counselor I was at work and I started to get weaker and sicker until by evening I thought I might be dying. I called the counselor who had Dr. Platt call me back immediately. Dr. Platt reassured me that it was just my body going through a detoxification process from sugar and caffeine. He said I'd be a lot better the next day, and sure enough, he was right.

I continue to go into Dr. Platt's office once a week. When I go in they check my blood pressure and my urine to see how much fat I am burning. They weigh me and I get a B12 shot.

It's been easy to stay on the diet and I've lost 60 pounds. Today I don't wake up with headaches any more—a miracle! My diarrhea's gone, no headaches, no asthma, and I have energy now. People tell me all the time that I look slimmer.

I really believe that the natural hormones have helped me the most. I'm able to control my eating now because I understand when and why I get hungry. Candy and caffeine just don't seem important to me anymore. I'm also not scared of getting out of control when I get to my goal weight. I used to be afraid of reaching my goal weight, thinking I would just gain it all back and then some, just like before. I now rely on the nutritional counselors at Dr. Platt's office because they always have good advice for me. They remind me that I'm going to be introducing carbohydrates one at a time, slowly, and that they will monitor the effects on me. I haven't reached my goal weight yet, but I already feel successful.

CHILDBIRTH AND HEADACHES

Shirley's headaches began after she gave birth to her first child. That's because pregnancy and birth cause vast hormonal shifts in some women. Hormones affect every aspect of pregnancy. The most obvious examples are women with low progesterone and high estrogen suffering from morning sickness and miscarriages.

By the time a woman reaches her third trimester, her placenta begins producing copious quantities of progesterone. Progesterone is the feel-good hormone and that's why the cliché has emerged of the "radiant" expectant mother nearing childbirth. Unfortunately, after a woman delivers, her progesterone level suddenly plummets. At this point the cliché reverses itself: post-partum depression is a common occurrence. What happened with Shirley was that her normally low progesterone levels sank even further after she gave birth, bringing on the headaches.

She'd already had symptoms of asthma as a result of her low progesterone and naturally those symptoms got worse after the birth of her child. Shirley reports feeling that her asthma got worse as her weight increased. This is not surprising, since the most likely cause of her asthma was a high estrogen level associated with low progesterone. The more fat cells a person has, the higher the estrogen levels. This, by the way, is the reason for the higher incidence of breast cancer in obese women.

Her feeling that it was harder and harder to control her weight through dieting as she aged is something everyone can identify with. People in their 40s often become alarmed at how stubbornly fat clings to their bodies. Throughout their teens, 20s and 30s they had been able to force themselves to shed a few pounds when they got desperate enough, but now nothing seems to work.

In Shirley's case, this was doubly true because she was over-producing insulin. Anyone who responds well to a high-protein diet is overproducing insulin. The most common reason why people overproduce insulin is that they are not producing enough progesterone, and as we get older progesterone levels decrease. This means that in middle age our bodies will produce more insulin. And insulin, as I've said again and again, is the fat-storing hormone.

SIGNS OF ESTROGEN DOMINANCE

Shirley's medical profile told me in many different ways that she was suffering from estrogen dominance. Very often, trouble with one's gall bladder is a complication of estrogen dominance. A hysterectomy tells me she had had fibroid tumors or another reproductive malady caused by estrogen. Her pear-shaped body type is the classic body type for someone overproducing estrogen.

MERIDIA FOR WEIGHT LOSS?—A FOOL'S ERRAND

Shirley was prescribed Meridia to help her lose weight. This was an error. Meridia is, in most cases, completely ineffective for weight loss.

Meridia is a combination of an SSRI (selective serotonin reuptake inhibitor) and an NRI (norepinephrine reuptake inhibitor). It was originally developed as an anti-depressant. When Phen/Fen was taken off the market, the manufacturers of Meridia decided to promote it for weight loss because Meridia affects the same neurotransrnitters that are were affected by Phen/Fen.

When the manufacturers of Meridia initially tried to get it through the FDA, it was rejected. It caused too many problems with elevated blood pressure. So they cut the dosage in half to reduce the blood pressure problem. Needless to say, Meridia's effectiveness for weight loss went down as well.

The whole approach to weight loss in conventional medicine has been predicated on the theory that people eat too much and that's why they have a weight problem. The medical community has been remiss in not addressing the true factors that cause weight gain.

Meridia might be of benefit in maintaining weight loss because it can reduce severe cravings for food. However, it does not address getting rid of fat. The great majority of overweight people have hormone problems: too much insulin, too much estrogen, an under active thyroid, etc. They will not be able to start burning fat until their hormones have been adjusted.

And as we get older, progesterone levels decrease. This means that in middle age our bodies will produce more insulin. And insulin, as I've said again and again, is the fat-storing hormone.

PREMARIN/PROVERA—DOCTOR'S FAVORITES

Shirley confesses that when she challenged her doctor about prescribing Premarin, she was chided for doing so. This is very common. Premarin is one of the largest-selling estrogen preparations in the world. Estrogen is the one hormone gynecologists know about and believe in, and Premarin is a formulation they're very familiar with. It's very common for gynecologists to look askance at any attempt to question Premarin's effectiveness.

I have had patients come back to me and report that

their doctors *forbade* them to take the natural progesterone I had prescribed. And the doctors would sternly insist these women continue their estrogen replacement therapy. I've heard of doctors who told women to throw their progesterone in the trash. These doctors are adamant about their love of estrogen.

Some time ago, I had a 59-year-old woman in my office. When she was 52 she was started on Premarin and Provera. By age 58 she had contracted breast cancer and they removed both breasts. The doctors then prescribed what was called an Estring, which is a high dose of estradiol [one of the three types of estrogen] inserted vaginally. So now she had estrogen sitting right next to her uterus. Now keep in mind that estrogen is the only known cause of cancer of the uterus.

This woman's sister had had cancer of the uterus. We're talking here about a woman who's genetically predisposed to contracting cancer of the uterus. So the patient is sitting there in my office and she tells me that she's due to have another Estring put in, as she has to have a new Estring inserted every two months. And her husband is sitting right next to her. And she's arguing with me about how she wants to have that Estring put back in. I asked her, "Why would you want to do that?" She replied that two gynecologists had told her that it's safe to do this.

I was dumbfounded. I said, "You've already donated both breasts, you want to give them your uterus as well?" Her husband couldn't believe her either. But women have been brainwashed as to the purported benefits of estrogen.

Provera is just as harmful as estrogen. It is a synthetic progestin and although it's chemical name is *medroxy progesterone* it has no relationship to natural, bio-identical progesterone. Many doctors mistakenly think Provera is the same as "progesterone." Provera is damaging to blood vessels (like estrogen), is lipogenic (it creates fat just like estrogen), and also increases a woman's chance of getting breast cancer (just like estrogen). However, in most cases it does prevent uterine cancer, which is why it is used in women taking Premarin who still have a uterus.

HORMONE RECEPTOR SITES

Hormones travel through the bloodstream in minute quantities. When they reach a receptor site that fits them, they attach to it and are able to influence the cell they have attached to. When a woman is estrogen dominant, i.e., has high estrogen and low progesterone, she may have completely different symptoms from another woman who is also estrogen dominant, because of different receptor sites.

Shirley developed asthma in her teenage years, a common problem induced by estrogen, not only in women but in men as well. Her asthma got worse as she got older, for several reasons. Her progesterone levels were retreating and very likely her estrogen levels may have been going up, as she got fatter. Fat cells produce estrogen. As previously stated, this may explain, at least in part, why obese women are more prone to breast cancer than women of normal weight.

Shirley also had estrogen receptor sites in her temporal arteries, explaining her migraine headaches. Many women have excess receptor sites in the uterus and breasts, creating severe menstrual cramps and breast tenderness during their periods. Later on, this intense stimulation leads to uterine fibroids or endometriosis, fibrocystic disease of the breasts or ovaries, and can result in uterine, ovarian, and breast cancer. None of these conditions occur when the body has enough natural progesterone to prevent them.

In addition, Shirley had described herself as having a

pear-shaped figure. This situation is found when the body is producing an overabundance of two different hormones—insulin and estrogen. Insulin puts fat on around the waist, and estrogen puts fat on around the hips, buttocks and thighs. This is true for both men and women. People with excesses of insulin and estrogen often have gall bladder problems as well.

TAKING THE TIME TO LISTEN

To this day Shirley remains angry about how she was treated by the medical establishment. This is not unusual. Many of my patients tell me horror stories about being patronized and not listened to. Until there is a change in doctor's attitudes, patients will continue to be misdiagnosed, with only their symptoms being addressed instead of the underlying causes of their illnesses. Doctors have to go back to listening to patients. There is no substitute for it.

Shirley was obviously hormonally challenged. A basic knowledge of natural hormones would have allowed her to eliminate her asthma which would have delighted her, to eliminate her headaches, which would have amazed her, and to get rid of her fat, which would have pleased her.

Needless to say, the use of bio-identical hormones for her was nothing short of miraculous.

CHAPTER 19

HUMAN GROWTH HORMONE (HGH)

A hormone I have not mentioned until now is human growth hormone (HGH). It regulates how the body grows, repairs itself and burns fat.

Interest in HGH replacement therapy has been growing ever since the publication of an article in the *New England Journal of Medicine* that showed HGH's rejuvenating potential. Daniel Rudman, M.D. documented the effects of six months of HGH supplementation upon 21 men aged 61 to 81 years. The results were remarkable. Every area measured improved—their body fat decreased, their lean body mass increased, their skin became thicker and their bone density increased. He said it was equivalent to undoing 10-20 years of aging.

Now dubbed the fountain of youth hormone, HGH has become a star feature at anti-aging clinics around the country. Today more people are being exposed to HGH than ever before, and it may be of possible benefit when used correctly.

However, as with any hormone, you must weigh the benefits against the risks. The primary role of HGH after age 30 is to help the body repair tissues—your growth stage is over. Giving a hormone that can promote the growth of tissue in high dosages may lead to unwanted side effects: acromegaly (enlargement of bony tissue); enlargement of the heart, leading to congestive heart failure; carpal tunnel syndrome, and arthritis. As people get older, they always have the possibility of cancerous tissue sitting somewhere in their bodies. HGH could stimulate the growth of that tissue. (Note that when HGH is used in children to stimulate normal levels of growth it doubles their chances of getting childhood leukemia.) HGH is not recommended for people with diabetes.

HGH is the main hormone put out by the pituitary gland. Using inappropriately high doses, especially over prolonged periods, can suppress the pituitary gland. It's the master gland, which can affect all other endocrine glands in the body, and create even more problems.

Another thing to keep in mind is that there are ways of elevating HGH levels without giving HGH directly. It can be done through the manipulation of other hormones, or by giving supplements called secretogues that stimulate HGH production. This is a much less expensive approach than the usual $1,500 to $3,000 price tag charged by many anti-aging clinics for HGH injections.

I have a lot of respect for nature. It seems to know what it's doing. When using hormones to alter the natural pattern, one must always be careful to approach it from a logical standpoint. Giving high dosages of HGH at a time when the body no longer needs high levels may be problematic.

It's the same with estrogen replacement. A woman never stops making estrogen. It is made in fat cells, skin cells and the adrenal glands, etc. The only need for the high levels given in HRT is if a woman is trying to get pregnant—not a likely scenario in menopausal women. This is another situation in which apparent benefits may be far outweighed by risks.

One last thought to keep in mind. There is a lot of interest in anti-aging remedies, which is the main reason for the use of HGH. HGH stimulates the production of IGF-1 (insulin-like growth factor-1) in the liver. Levels of IGF-1 are used to monitor HGH production. There are recent studies that indicate that IGF-1 may actually speed up the aging process and it is considered the number two hormone to do this. Insulin, by the way, is number one.

Another concern is that they find high levels of IGF-1 in the cancerous tissues of people with breast and prostate cancer. My feeling is that the jury is still out when it comes to using HGH. It may possibly be administered safely with carefully controlled dosages and monitoring for untoward effects: edema, tingling in the fingertips, arthritic pains, and unwanted growths. However, the bottom line to the use of HGH is that it may be illegal to prescribe it. Congress passed a law years ago addressing the off-label use of HGH, stating that it is illegal to use it as an anti-aging drug or for other unsupported claims.

CHAPTER 20

MARGARET O.—BATTLING THE MEDICAL ESTABLISHMENT

Margaret O. is a well-educated woman, an accomplished musician and a teacher. She came to me at the age of 67 having spent the previous 37 years seeking the solution to a serious weight problem. She had been a size 22 for most of her adult life, even though she was physically active and ate healthy foods in reasonable quantities. But she had a hormonal profile that made her body store fat.

I want you to hear her story because I see so many women

like her: well-educated, inquisitive, avid readers who study
health and medicine in an attempt to understand their own
bodies. Their weight problem isn't their fault, but the medical
establishment thwarts their honest efforts to break through
their difficulties.

When I started gaining weight in my 30s I wanted to find out
why. I wasn't eating any more than I had been before the weight gain
and my level of physical activity was the same. Instinctively I knew
some other variable was at work here. At first I went to the doctors at
Kaiser Hospital where I have my medical plan. I thought they could
help me.

They did a series of tests on me and declared that I had an under
active thyroid. That made sense to me and I was hopeful that with thy-
roid medication my metabolism could be ratcheted up and my weight
would start to go down. They prescribed the thyroid hormone
Synthroid. I took it but nothing happened.

So I went back to Kaiser and told them I was still gaining weight.
They gave me the same tests over again and they gave me another pre-
scription for Synthroid. It seems this was the only thing they knew.
When I went back a third time and told them I wasn't getting any
results they just looked at me strangely and told me to eat less.

From this experience I learned to harbor a healthy skepticism
about the medical profession. Today I seek my own conclusions and I
don't take things at face value any more. Being an educated person, I
began reading everything I could about how the body metabolizes food.
Meanwhile, I tried every diet that came down the pike. I tried
Optifast, Shaklee and many other diets. I would lose weight on each of
these, but I never lost fat—always muscle. I would look at myself in
the mirror after each of these diets and see flesh just hanging on me.
The diets were hard to stay on and they made me weak. I remember one
time about six years ago, I was on a vacation in Hawaii after com-
pleting a diet that consisted of eating nothing but protein drinks four
times a day. There I was, hiking along this trail, and when our group

*came to a small fissure on the trail everyone leapt across it. But I could-
n't get my body to do it. I was that weak. Every time I came off one of
those diets I gained back more than I had weighed before. This went
on for my entire adulthood. I got up to 240 pounds and I am only 5'1"
tall. It became hard to move around and hard to go shopping. Clothes
were a problem, so I either sewed or bought them from Nordstrom cat-
alog. I was a size 22. One doesn't find beautiful clothing in those sizes.
The simple act of getting up from a chair or a sofa was hard for me.
So was going to a restaurant and sitting in a booth. I never knew
whether I could fit into the booth.*

*I went on like this for 37 years, seeking answers, talking to peo-
ple, trying diets and joining support groups. Many times I got tired of
searching and just let myself go. But even when I'd given up and gotten sloppy again there was always part of my mind sort of passively
available, listening, waiting to find out about something that might
make permanent weight loss possible.*

*My first break came during menopause, when I read Dr. John R.
Lee's "What Your Doctor May Not Tell You about Menopause." This
book had a lot of inside-track information about hormone replacement
therapy. It gave me information about hormones that I had been seeking all my life. Dr. Lee was the first doctor to come out saying that
Premarin and all the synthetic estrogen hormones being given to women
at menopause were actually hurting them. He talked about how estrogen made the body store fat. I thought: At last! A clue! I began to
believe that I had a hormone problem, one that went beyond my under
active thyroid.*

*But I needed more specific information and I needed a doctor who
could help me balance my hormones. I went to the endocrinologists at
Kaiser but that was a lost cause. They wanted to get me on Premarin
as fast as they could! They are part of that medical establishment Dr.
Lee writes about that is brainwashed about Premarin. They certainly
were not about to help me.*

I knew I needed to find an endocrinologist outside the Kaiser system who agreed with Dr. Lee's ideas and was ready to buck the whole system regarding Premarin. But where do you find someone like that? My entire life's experience had taught me that doctors were, for the most part, like Stepford wives. They were cheerleaders for a system that reduced reality to a few simple clichés. I was also leery of exposing myself to more insults from doctors. Whenever I would go in for these consultations about my weight, I could see exactly what these doctors were thinking. Whether they said it or not, they gave me the feeling they thought I was some kind of binge eater looking for a shortcut or a miracle.

I started feeling trapped; I had that discouraged, sort of Kafkaesque sensation like I'd gotten back in my 30s.

But then over New Year's my husband and I were at our condo in the desert and I saw Dr. Platt on television. Everything he said made so much sense that I made an appointment to see him!

I brought my Kaiser folder to Dr. Platt and he did a battery of hormone tests. I found him easy to talk to. He also had me consult with one of his nutritionists. At first I was cynical about talking to another nutritionist. I have been through a lot of nutrition classes sponsored by Kaiser. That's another insulting thing they do when you are looking for help with weight loss: they make you take these classes. I've been through umpteen nutrition classes and cholesterol classes and so forth. You name it and Kaiser wants to put you through it.

But I found Dr. Platt's people different. They really have knowledge that helps you and a way of sharing it that I understood.

Dr. Platt told me that when I lost weight my cholesterol would go down. My cholesterol was 293 when I went in there. Kaiser had wanted me to take Zocor for my high cholesterol, which is one of about three or four statin drugs on the market. But I said no. Dr. Platt and I are working on my cholesterol with niacin. Within the first two months of starting with Dr. Platt, my cholesterol dropped 50 points.

When the hormone tests came back, Dr. Platt and I sat down and went over them. My low thyroid was still there and Dr. Platt adjusted my thyroid giving me T3 in addition to T4. He explained to me why the Synthroid by itself wasn't helping me. It made me angry to think I had been faithfully taking this stuff for 20 years and it had been doing nothing for me.

As I lost weight I gained energy. It became easier to do just about anything. So far I've lost 38 pounds. I weigh 202 now. But I'm wearing a size 16 and there's no flab! I used to feel impaired, but I'm not impaired anymore. I have no problems getting up off of the sofa or in and out of a booth.

I've always been an active person even when it was a struggle to move around. I still work in a gift shop every day, sing in a choir, volunteer at my Temple, teach piano privately at home and cook with my husband every night. My ideal weight is 141. I am confident I will get there.

NEAR MISSES

Over the years I've seen a lot of patients like Margaret, very smart people who try to approach their weight problems intelligently but still can't lose weight. I find them especially poignant. With all of their reading and detective work, they're nonetheless thwarted by our popular culture of dieting and our uninformed medical system. Margaret made some good inroads, but she just didn't take the right path to get to where she wanted to go. She had read Dr. Lee and understood the value of natural progesterone. Unfortunately, the type of progesterone he promotes does not have a high enough strength. He recommends the over-the-counter type of progesterone, which is 20 milligrams, and a woman generally needs about 200 milligrams a day.

Margaret also suspected that she had a thyroid problem and

even her doctors determined that it was true. But they placed her on the wrong thyroid medication. This is extremely common, as you've already seen with Brenda J. and Rhonda Y. She was given the T4 hormone Synthroid when what she also needed was T3. That's the most common error made by conventional doctors when treating overweight people with under active thyroid glands. They don't realize that people can have normal levels of T4 and still be hypothyroid. Few doctors look at a patient's T3 levels, T3 being the active hormone that regulates metabolism. The logical question here is: Why don't doctors start looking at T3 levels so they can cover all the bases for their patients suffering from hypothyroidism? Or, put another way, why does it seem as though doctors sabotage people like Margaret?

YO-YO DIETING AND WEIGHT LOSS

Margaret is the type of person who has the most difficult time losing weight. Her long history of repeated diets had turned her body into an extremely efficient, sophisticated, fat-storing machine.

The body does not know about weight loss—it only understands the threat of starvation. Its main concern is survival. When insufficient quantities of fuel are consumed, it naturally thinks that it may be facing starvation. It begins to create and store fat in a highly efficient manner.

This is an important point and bears repeating. It is important for people interested in losing weight to understand how their body operates. The body likes fat. It likes to create it, hold onto it and does not like to burn it.

When people go on starvation weight loss programs, most of the weight loss that occurs is from muscle loss—the body will not bum burn fat when it is starving. Muscle weighs three times as much as fat, so people can get a rapid weight loss, which makes them happy. This happiness, unfortunately, is short-lived because there is a rapid regaining. Less muscle tissue means less room for carbohydrate (sugar) storage, so any excess is apt to be stored in the fat cells. And less muscle means less fat-burning tissue, since muscle is the fat-burning tissue of the body.

Added to this, the body becomes even more efficient at storing fat. The bottom line: cutting calories is probably not the best weight loss approach for long-term weight management.

Fat is a very efficient fuel—it burns at nine calories per gram—and the body wisely reserves its most efficient fuel for last. A good example of this is Karen Carpenter, the singer who died of anorexia nervosa. This was a woman who placed her body in a continuous state of starvation. When they did her autopsy, they discovered she had almost no heart muscle. Her body had eaten its most vital organ rather than give up its last ounce of fat.

A MORE ENLIGHTENED APPROACH

Could anyone have been more proactive, determined and methodical in her search for weight management than Margaret? And yet her search went on, unsuccessfully, for 37 years. That's how difficult it is to get help with obesity in this culture! It is time to change our assumptions about why people's bodies store fat. And it's time to give patients a more enlightened and helpful approach to weight loss.

CHAPTER 21

MENOPAUSE and PERIMENOPAUSE

I have purposefully put this chapter towards the end of the book, even though, for many readers, it will be the most important. If you have gone through the preceding chapters you should now have a feeling of the importance of hormones: how necessary it is for them to be in balance, and the devastating consequences that occur when they are out of balance.

You should also be aware of the tragic lack of knowledge that many doctors have regarding how the body operates, especially with regard to hormones. It is no wonder that the approach to the menopause in women and the andropause in men has been basically unchanged for the last 50 years. This lack of knowledge represents more than an inconvenience to women and men in terms of their symptoms; it has literally put their health at risk for serious diseases and higher death rates. This particularly relates to two problems: the lack of knowledge for preventing many of the diseases of aging using natural hormones, and how the incorrect use of hormones can cause unnecessary deaths due to cancer, heart disease, and strokes.

USING BIO-IDENTICAL HORMONES

Perhaps the most commonly known application of hormone therapy is in the treatment of women going through the menopause. The term "menopause" means the absence of periods, whether it be naturally occurring or surgically-induced (i.e. hysterectomy).

As women approach the time of menopause, the perimenopause, there is a drop in hormones produced by the ovaries, which can produce a number of symptoms. The most common symptom is the onset of irregular periods, perhaps occurring sporadically and of shorter than usual duration. This reflects a drop in estrogen levels. At the same time, a drop in progesterone levels may cause women to experience an increase in PMS or cramps, a drop in libido, an increase in weight and more difficulty in thinking.

Eventually, estrogen and progesterone levels will fall to a level where they can no longer prepare the uterus for bleeding—the menopause has begun.

Some women go through this period of their lives with little or no symptoms. Other women develop hot flashes, night sweats, etc., and become very uncomfortable.

But no matter how you look at it, the menopause is a very natural condition that all women eventually go through. The problem is that the medical system has taken this natural condition and turned it into a disease that has to be treated.

Back in the 1960's, Robert Wilson, M.D., a gynecologist in New York City, published a book called "Feminine Forever." He stated that when women go through the menopause, "they enter a 'vapid cow-like state' and became very unpleasant companions for their husbands." It was for the benefit of the husbands that he felt women should be treated, not for themselves. He received tremendous financial backing from the makers of Premarin, who helped publish his book and sent him on a nation-wide tour so that he could promote Premarin to physicians.

Eventually, Premarin became the largest selling drug in the world. However, a darker side to hormone replacement therapy began to emerge. In the first 10 years of use, it is estimated that somewhere between 200,000 and 2,000,000 women developed cancer of the uterus. Instead of removing it from the market, they added Provera to it. Although this reduced the risk of uterine cancer, it quadrupled a woman's chances of getting breast cancer from the estrogen.

Along the way they started ascribing certain benefits to hormone therapy with estrogen without the means to back up their claims.

They claimed that estrogen was beneficial for osteoporosis, and yet no study has shown estrogen to reverse osteoporosis. In 1999, the FDA finally took away osteoporosis as an indication to use estrogen. However, in all fairness, I should say that estrogen can help delay the onset of osteoporosis, at least temporarily. They also claimed that estrogen was good for the heart. However, every long-term study of estrogen has indicated that it causes an increase in the incidence of heart attacks and strokes. It is contra-indicated in coronary artery disease and cerebrovascular disease, so I fail to see the claimed benefit of estrogen in these conditions.

In order to decide once and for all the benefits of long-term treatment with estrogen, the largest study ever of hormone replacement therapy was conducted. It was called "The Women's Health Initiative," and involved about 162,000 women. It was proposed as an eight year study to monitor women on Premarin/Provera therapy or Premarin by itself for those women who did not have a uterus.

Two years into the study they started getting some alarming statistics, but, they continued with the study. However, after 5½ years they felt ethically they could not continue. There were a significantly higher number of women with aggressive-type breast cancers along with a higher incidence of cardiovascular complications.

In the summer of 2002, the Premarin/Provera arm of the study was halted. It was front page news in every newspaper in America; it was the cover story of all news magazines and became fodder for TV news programs and talk shows.

For the first time in history, women were made aware of the truth that had been known for 30 years, that estrogen might not be safe.

The consistent recommendation was—go talk to your health care practitioner. However, if doctors were aware of the prior studies done in the 1990's, they might not have started these drugs in the first place. The physician's usual response to women's concerns about the study included: don't worry about it, or the benefits outweigh the risk (they don't), or it's your decision.

The other arm of the study, Premarin by itself, was stopped in March of 2004—again, risks outweighed potential benefits.

Into this wasteland of no knowledge about hormones, walked Suzanne Somers. With her book called *The Sexy Years*, Ms. Somers propelled herself into the position of being the new guru of hormone replacement therapy.

Her book demonstrated some amazingly positive attributes. For the first time in history, women were made aware of "bio-identical hormones"—hormones that were chemically identical to their own and could be obtained from compound pharmacies.

No longer did they have to subject themselves to synthetic drugs that mimicked hormones, nor did they have to take hormones appropriate for horses rather than humans.

Another tremendous benefit of her book was the insistence that women have to become pro-active about their health; they cannot rely on the traditional medical system to keep them healthy.

However, there are some points that she has made in her book that I feel require some clarification.

First off, just because a hormone is "bio-identical" does not necessarily mean that it is safe. Hormones are extremely potent chemicals and must be used judiciously. Some of the doctors that Ms. Somers interviewed are very strong proponents of estrogen. She quotes one doctor as stating that the only time a woman is healthy is when she is having her periods. To achieve this aim, this doctor provides her patients with exceptionally high levels of estrogen in order to have them re-start menstruation. She has patients in their 80's and 90's bleeding every month and bent over with menstrual cramps. These women, needless to say, are intentionally put into the dangerous position of estrogen-dominance.

In my own practice, the sickest women I have ever seen are those that had been estrogen-dominant, or were estrogen-dominant when I first met them.

Let me remind you that anytime you utilize either a hormone or a drug, you have to weigh the benefits vs. the risks. I look at estrogen as primarily being a toxic hormone. It is known to cause six different cancers in women: breast, uterine, ovarian, cervical, vaginal and colon cancer. It may cause Alzheimer's disease, strokes, heart attacks, and phlebitis with fatal pulmonary emboli. It may cause fibroids, endometriosis, adhesions, fibrocystic disease, asthma, migraine headaches and gallbladder disease.

Estrogen is the hormone that causes women to experience menstrual cramps, PMS, breast tenderness, and nausea when they are pregnant. To add insult to injury, estrogen is lipogenic. It creates fat around the hips, thighs and buttocks, and it is the cause of cellulite.

Try telling women with a number of these problems that they are healthy because they are having periods and you might get an argument from them.

It is surprising that Suzanne Somers, who had already had estrogen-induced breast cancer (she used to call estrogen her "happy pills") is now proposing that women take what I consider exceedingly high levels of estrogen. Not a week goes by that I do not have a patient who has had an estrogen-induced cancer while they were still having their periods. In other words, their own estrogen caused these cancers—it does not get more 'bio-identical' than your own hormones.

Interestingly, every problem, every complication, every downside to estrogen is eliminated by another hormone called progesterone (this is not to be confused with medroxyprogesterone, also known as Provera—a synthetic chemical having no relationship to natural progesterone.) Anytime there are high levels of estrogen, such as those proposed by the book, "The Sexy Years," there must be a sufficient amount of progesterone to be protective. I believe the levels of progesterone recommended in her book are woefully inadequate and inappropriately administered.

I will be giving my advice on the proper dosing in chapter 22. Keep in mind several factors:

1. Women never stop making estrogen—it is probably the only hormone that never has to be replaced. It is made by fat cells, skin cells and the adrenal glands.

2. Women stop making progesterone. Because of this, they are always at risk for developing breast cancer, uterine cancer, ovarian cancer and colon cancer, etc. from estrogen.

BACK TO THE MENOPAUSE

When certain hormone levels decrease, for either natural or surgical reasons, the pituitary responds by putting out certain hormones of its own to stimulate the ovaries to make more hormones. The pituitary and hypothalamus glands are the areas of the brain that control other glands throughout the body. In this case, the pituitary puts out a hormone called luteinizing hormone (LH) to stimulate the ovaries to make more hormones. It is felt that LH is the primary cause of the vascular symptoms women experience when going through the menopausal period—hot flashes and night sweats.

It is my feeling that the primary reason the pituitary has for trying to raise ovarian hormone levels is so the woman can get pregnant. Once the pituitary is convinced a woman no longer needs to procreate, it stops sending out the signals and the hot flashes, etc. disappear. However, once a woman is placed on high levels of hormone replacement therapy, the pituitary gets confused. Now it is convinced the woman is trying to get pregnant and so whenever there is a significant drop (i.e. stopping Premarin, etc.) the symptoms recur.

MY APPROACH

There are certain things that have to be taken into consideration. Every woman is different; there is no one-size-fits-all approach when using hormones.

The ovaries put out four different hormones—estrogen, progesterone, testosterone and DHEA. Replacement of any or all of these hormones can alleviate symptoms. The primary aim of the replacement of hormones is to keep people healthy and to prevent the body from deteriorating.

Since I look at estrogen as a potentially toxic and fat-creating hormone, and since the body never stops making estrogen, I utilize a relatively sparing approach to its use. I will primarily use estrogen for several reasons—to help alleviate hot flashes or night sweats, to help with "brain fog," and to relieve vaginal dryness. I will be discussing dosages, along with the various types of natural bio-identical estrogen available, in a later chapter. When women enter the menopause they stop making progesterone. Prior to the menopause their progesterone levels are dropping, which causes women to experience an increase in PMS, breast tenderness and cramps, etc. They might notice the development of fibroids or fibrocystic disease in the breast, both conditions caused by estrogen when there is not enough progesterone to protect them.

Progesterone is one of the most important hormones in a woman's body and is probably the only hormone that has to be replaced after the menopause.

THE BENEFITS OF PROGESTERONE

Throughout the book, I have presented a number of patients who had various medical problems. Every one of them had conditions related to a deficiency of progesterone. Keep in mind that every problem related to estrogen is created by a progesterone deficiency. Giving women natural progesterone takes away menstrual cramps, PMS, breast tenderness, menstrual migraines and asthma. It prevents fibroids, endometriosis, fibrocystic disease and estrogen-induced cancers.

The benefits of progesterone after the menopause are as follows: it can eliminate hot flashes and prevent and treat osteoporosis. It is a natural anti-depressant, the feel-good hormone for women. Progesterone is thermogenic—it helps fat to burn. It prevents Alzheimer's disease, is great for the heart and restores the libido (estrogen does nothing for the libido).

Throughout the book are numerous references to the benefits of this hormone in terms of preventing estrogen-induced cancer. It helps eliminate Attention Deficit Disorder (ADD) and is the number one hormone for lowering insulin levels, thereby helping to prevent obesity and adult-onset diabetes.

WHAT ABOUT TESTOSTERONE?

The ovaries are the primary (but not the only source) of testosterone. My feeling is that testosterone is the 2nd most important hormone to be replaced after progesterone. Again, it certainly is a lot more important than estrogen. In women, testosterone is the main hormone that prevents Alzheimer's (progesterone is 2nd). It is the number one hormone for preventing and treating osteoporosis (progesterone is 2nd). It is the number one hormone for the heart because there are more testosterone receptor sites in heart muscle than in any other tissue (250,000 people die of congestive heart failure every year, caused by weakening of the heart muscle). You cannot build muscle without testosterone, so it helps keep muscles toned; it gives women more energy and makes them feel more assertive. Testosterone is also necessary for an interest in sex;

women started on testosterone and progesterone often start fantasizing in about 6 weeks.

Another benefit of testosterone is that it can, when used correctly, eliminate urinary incontinence in about six days. I will be going over the correct dosages in a later chapter.

DHEA—THE ANTI AGING HORMONE

In the teenage years, dehydroepiendosterone (DHEA) is the most abundant hormone in the body. As time goes on, the levels go down. It is looked at as the biological marker for aging: those people with the highest levels seem to have the greatest longevity. Forty percent of DHEA is produced by the ovaries; the other 60% comes mainly from the adrenals. It is a hormone that helps to control the immune system and helps to prevent cancer, heart disease and arthritis. Women with the highest levels of DHEA have the lowest incidence of breast cancer. DHEA helps to prevent the "bad" cholesterol (LDL) from oxidizing. It is a precursor to estrogen and testosterone, so it can help to alleviate hot flashes. It is also considered a fat-burning hormone.

Surprisingly, even though it is a very powerful hormone, it can be purchased over the counter as a food supplement in drug and health food stores. This by itself is a testament to the lack of information that doctors have about hormones. Like any other hormone, it should be used correctly, and only if there is a deficiency.

CHAPTER 22

ANDROPAUSE: THE MALE MENOPAUSE

An often over-looked fact is that men and women produce exactly the same hormones. As is the case in women, most hormone levels become lower in men as they get older. Since hormones affect every system of the body, there are profound changes that occur as one ages.

Interestingly, it is more important for men to receive bio-identical hormone replacement than it is for women. The consequences of altered hormone levels in men may lead to coronary artery disease, Alzheimer's disease, prostate cancer, osteoporosis, depression, and other diseases.

TESTOSTERONE

Unquestionably, the most important hormone to be considered for replacement is testosterone. It is most often thought of as a sex hormone, and it is, but it has other functions that are probably more vital.

It is the main hormone for the prevention of Alzheimer's disease. Studies done by the National Institutes of Health have confirmed this.

It is the number one hormone affecting heart tissue, including the coronary arteries, the conduction system and, most important, the heart muscle itself. There are more testosterone receptor sites in heart muscle than in any other muscle in the body. Two studies came out in 2003 demonstrating the use of testosterone in men with massive heart attacks. This is a situation that almost always results in the occurrence of congestive heart failure (CHF), a weakening of the heart muscle resulting in the backup of fluid into the lungs and possibly the rest of the body. Those groups of men who received testosterone failed to develop CHF; the other group all went into failure.

The development of osteoporosis, although not as common in men as women, actually has more dire consequences. A fractured hip in a male, most commonly related to osteoporosis, is associated with a 25% mortality rate in the first year of occurrence. Testosterone prevents and reverses osteoporosis.

An extremely common consequence of low testosterone levels in men is the onset of depression. They lose their interest in life, their vigor, their *joi de vivre*, and their energy levels go down. Replacement of testosterone in these situations brings back energy, restores lost strength and an interest in life, and leads to the buildup of muscle.

Very often the libido returns. I've had male patients in their 70's that hadn't had sex in 25 years who are now having sex on a daily basis. Of course, their partner's hormones had to be dealt with as well.

THE CORRECT USE OF TESTOSTERONE

As with any other hormone, testosterone must be used correctly. Testosterone can convert into other hormones, which can create problems—this will be covered later in the chapter.

It is often beneficial to have blood levels of testosterone determined. The most important test in this regard would be a free testosterone level, not the more frequently determined total testosterone level. The free testosterone level determines the biologically active testosterone that is available. However, levels of testosterone go up and down during the day.

The highest levels occur early in the morning, before testing is usually done. I have found that most men after the age of 50 will either have a level below the normal range or else in the lower range of normal. And yet, many of these men will still be getting morning erections (an excellent indication of adequate testosterone levels) and have no problems with performance or libido.

No matter how low the level, if a man has no sexual problems I do not replace testosterone. Normal levels of free testosterone range from 50 to 210. Levels of total testosterone range from 250 to 1,000. I find levels of testosterone more useful in determining correct replacement dosages—too much or too little.

When replacing testosterone, one should be aware that this hormone can be converted into other hormones that may have unpleasant consequences. One is estrogen, which can cause prostate cancer and possibly colon cancer, and the other is dihydrotestosterone (DHT), which may cause prostate enlargement and male pattern hair loss.

Because of these possibilities, the level of these two hormones should be monitored. High levels of DHT can often be avoided by correct placement of testosterone cream or gel on the skin. It is always best to apply testosterone to areas of the body devoid of hair. There are certain enzymes found around hair follicles that can convert testosterone into DHT (in other words, shaving an area will not help.) These acceptable areas may include the upper and inner arm, shoulders, back of the knees and around the ankles. Certain supplements can also help in this regard, among them saw palmetto, beta-sitosterol and pygeum.

There are ways to keep estradiol levels lower. Discuss with the compound pharmacist or your medical doctor the addition of 10% chrysin to the testosterone cream—it is an aromatase inhibitor. Aromatase is necessary to convert testosterone into estrogen, so anything that lowers this enzyme is beneficial. Arimidex can also be used to lower estradiol. The recommended dose is 50 mcg per day, which must be compounded.

Zinc is another important supplement to use while on testosterone. The prostate gland absorbs more zinc than any other area of the body. Zinc also acts as an aromatase inhibitor, thereby keeping estrogen levels low. (Note: I use the words estradiol and estrogen interchangeably). As a side note, the eyes are second in the absorption of zinc, which is useful for the prevention of macular degeneration, the most common cause of adult blindness.

I will be discussing prostate cancer in a separate section. The dosage of testosterone should be about ¼ tsp. of a 10% transdermal cream twice a day. The prescription should read:

Testosterone 10%. Apply ¼ tsp BID to hairless area (upper, inner arm, shoulders, back of knees or ankles). When the libido returns, one dose a day may be adequate.

Blood tests that should be monitored include:

- Total testosterone

- Free testosterone

- Estradiol

- Dihydrotestosterone

- PSA with free PSA

The benefits of testosterone far outweigh any potential downside. But its use should be done safely with attention to prostate health. In addition, too much testosterone can raise cholesterol levels, cause male pattern baldness, raise levels of red blood cells and possibly cause aggressive behavior.

WHY PROGESTERONE

Most likely if you were to question your doctor about progesterone, his/her response would be, "It is a female hormone." As stated throughout the book, men and women have exactly the same hormones, but in different levels.

As men get older, their level of progesterone becomes lower. Around the age of 50, the levels become almost non-existent. This is about the same age that men start putting on their "middle-aged paunch." Could there be a connection?

The answer to this question is a most definite yes. And the reason: Progesterone is the number one hormone for lowering insulin levels, the hormone that creates fat right around the middle. This is also the time that men might be experiencing fatigue between 3 and 4 in the afternoon or getting sleepy while driving or after eating. These are the classic times related to over-production of insulin. When insulin levels go up, blood sugar goes down.

The brain deprived of sugar gets sleepy. The number one cause of people falling asleep while driving is hypoglycemia. The number one cause of hypoglycemia is too much insulin. The number one cause of too much insulin is low progesterone. One of the first benefits people experience after starting progesterone is they no longer get sleepy in the afternoon, after eating, or while driving.

Another reason for the replacement of progesterone relates to estrogen. The onset of the andropause primarily relates to the lowering of testosterone. As testosterone levels decrease, this is often associated with an increase in estrogen. I will be discussing estrogen in the sub-section on prostate cancer.

For now, let me just reiterate that progesterone helps to prevent every cancer caused by estrogen. Other benefits from progesterone in men are as follows: prevention of Alzheimer's disease, prevention of osteoporosis, prevention of coronary artery spasm, reversal of depression, and elimination of asthma.

The dramatic effects of progesterone in men are perhaps best illustrated by one of my patients, Jim B. When I first met Jim, he was 54 years old. He came into my office, sat down and with no other preamble stated, "Doc, if you don't help me, I'm going to commit suicide." He added that I was his last resort.

He had four major complaints: 1) he was obviously depressed, 2) he was severely hypoglycemic, 3) he had asthma and 4) he had osteoporosis.

I told him right off that his problems were easily resolved, and that he had a deficiency of progesterone. In response he looked at me quizzically and said that over the last several years he had been back and forth across the country, had spent tens of thousands of dollars, had consultations with the best doctors in the finest clinics and institutions, had hundreds of blood tests and procedures and no one had ever mentioned the word "progesterone," nor tested for it. And here, in the space of several minutes, I told him this was his problem.

Although he strongly suspected I was a "quack," he agreed to a trial of progesterone. In only three days he was saying, "In my entire life, I have never felt so good."

To me, this response was expected. Progesterone affects every neurotransmitter in the brain and can readily eliminate depression. This hormone prevents the over-production of insulin and helps hypoglycemia. Progesterone is wonderful for eliminating asthma. This may possibly be related to its anti-estrogen effect. Estrogen is a common cause of asthma and men often have high levels of estrogen. Progesterone is also beneficial for preventing and treating osteoporosis.

It is not surprising that every medical specialist he spoke to was unable to diagnose his problem. During their training, doctors receive an extremely limited knowledge of hormones and thereby are frequently unable to help patients get well.

I consider progesterone the second most important hormone for replacement in men. The prescription I recommend would be:

Progesterone 100 mg / ¼ tsp

¼ tsp BID for two weeks, then ¼ tsp QD

Progesterone is best applied to the wrist area and
    lower forearm.

Start off with ¼ tsp twice a day for two weeks, then
    ¼ tsp once a day.

There are actually no downsides to using this hormone. It must be obtained from a compound pharmacy. The cream is used in lieu of an oral form in order to bypass the liver.

I have only had one complaint from a male patient whom

I placed on progesterone. He said it made him too compassionate. Wives, are you listening?

In all fairness I should mention that this particular patient had ADHD. As I described in the chapter about ADHD these patients have high levels of adrenalin to combat their persistent hypoglycemia induced by high insulin levels. Adrenalin is the 'anger' hormone. By giving him progesterone, it lowered his insulin levels, he no longer had hypoglycemia, and he stopped pouring out adrenaline (i.e., he became compassionate).

Progesterone also eliminates restless leg syndrome (RLS), another condition caused by too much adrenaline, although this is not recognized by the medical community. Doctors claim there is no known cause for this condition and that it is incurable. They treat it with toxic anti-Parkinsonian drugs, once again treating symptoms instead of the cause. Use of progesterone often elimates RLS in about one week.

Adults with ADHD, RLS, fibromyalgia—all conditions associated with too much adrenaline—usually require progesterone three times a day, and must cut back on their carbohydrate intake to reduce sugar and insulin levels.

WHAT ABOUT DHEA?

DHEA is considered the biological marker for aging—people with the highest levels seem to have the greatest longevity. DHEA has its own receptor sites and seems to help in preventing cancer, heart disease, arthritis, osteoporosis and Alzheimer's. It also increases one's feeling of well-being. It raises growth hormone levels and breaks down into testosterone, which may possibly be the reason for some of these benefits.

The primary concern related to DHEA is that it can raise estradiol levels, the hormone related to prostate cancer and possibly colon cancer. However, given in correct dosages, this rarely happens. The concept of hormone replacement therapy is to replace what's missing. There are limited numbers of receptor sites available for each hormone, so extremely high doses can result in untoward happenings.

In replacing DHEA, correct blood levels must be obtained. The correct lab test should be: DHEA-S (not plain DHEA). Most men in their 50's have levels around 175 or less. My goal in replacing DHEA levels is to achieve levels that were present around the age of 40. This would be equal to a DHEA-S level of around 400-500. For those men with levels of less than 100, I give a dosage of 50mg a day. For levels higher than 100, I start with a 25 mg dosage.

Estradiol levels should be monitored while taking DHEA. Ideally, estradiol should not be higher than 20. If this level is higher than this to begin with, I do not give DHEA until the level is lowered. If the level goes over 40 while on DHEA, I cut back the dosage or the frequency of administration.

THOUGHTS ABOUT PROSTATE CANCER

Allowed a long enough life span, most men will develop prostate cancer. Statistically, only 7% of prostate cancers will metastasize. In essence, this means that if left alone, most men would die with prostate cancer and not from it.

Based on that information, it would appear logical to use watchful waiting as a feasible approach to prostate cancer. The diagnosis of this disease is done by sticking needles into the prostate. Is it possible that this actually causes some of theses cancers to metastasize by allowing cancer cells to get into the blood at the time of the biopsy?

The traditional thinking in medicine is that testosterone is the hormone that causes prostate cancer. And yet, men with the highest levels of testosterone have the lowest incidence of prostate cancer. And why wouldn't males at the age of 17 have prostate cancer, when the levels of testosterone are at their highest?

Around the age of 50, men's production of progesterone drops to very low levels. Starting in their 20's, men's level of testosterone starts dropping, becoming very low by the age of 60. While this is happening, the level of estradiol is rising. Men in their 50's and beyond almost always have higher levels of estrogen than women have.

Keep in mind that estrogen causes six different cancers in women. It is the only known cause of uterine cancer (except for the drug Tamoxifen). In the embryonic stage, the uterus and the prostate both arise from the same tissue. If estrogen is basically the only cause of uterine cancer, then is it possible that estrogen is the hormone that causes prostate cancer? Logically, it would appear to be so. Yet, in some cases, estrogen is used to treat prostate cancer.

Most of the attention in treating prostate cancer is to eliminate testosterone. Often the drug Lupron is administered, and many times it appears to be beneficial. However, it not only lowers testosterone levels, it also eliminates estradiol. Perhaps this is its main benefit.

I am a very strong advocate of preventive medicine, in a world where it just doesn't seem to exist.

Prostate cancer is probably a disease to be prevented rather than to be treated. Here is a list of some of the supplements known to prevent and/or treat prostate cancer:

Lycopene - 30 mg/day

Vitamin D - 2000 i.u./day

Vitamin E - 800 i.u./day in the form of mixed tocopherols

Selenium 200 mcg/day

Zinc - 25-50 mg/day

Indole-3-carbinol- 300 mg/day

Beta-sitosterol - 300 mg/day

For those men with elevated PSA levels, it is imperative to check the free PSA level. An elevated PSA is considered any level greater than 2.5 (not 4.0, as commonly thought). A free PSA is an important determinant of the possibility of cancer. Keep in mind that the most common cause of an elevated PSA level is benign prostatic hypertrophy (BPH). Another frequent cause is prostatitis (infectious or inflammatory).

A free PSA percentage greater than 20% suggests the absence of cancer; a level less than 10% suggests its presence. Levels from 11% to 20% are in the gray area.

My approach to patients with any elevation of PSA is to start progesterone (an anti-estrogen hormone), give those supplements previously listed, and follow the PSA and free PSA levels. This approach is my own. Any prostate concerns must be discussed with your own physician.

CHAPTER 23

WHAT DO I DO NOW? THE HOW-TO SECTION

The replacement of natural hormones is not an exact science. It requires a team approach among the patient, the doctor and the compound pharmacist.

Over time, dosages may have to be adjusted, based not so much on lab tests as on symptoms. As stated before, there is no one-size-fits-all dosage. Every person's hormone levels are different and they can even change during different hours of the day.

However, after the menopause, there are certain truisms: the estrogen level is lower but it is still being produced;

testosterone levels are much lower; DHEA levels are at least 40%-50% lower and progesterone levels are virtually nonexistent.

Dosages that I am recommending are based on feedback and experience with thousands of men and women that I have treated. Once you feel that a certain approach might be appropriate for yourself, make notes and discuss it with your doctor. If he/she feels comfortable with the suggestions, a prescription may be obtained that can only be provided by a compound pharmacy. These are regular pharmacies that also have pharmacists specially trained in compounding various pharmaceuticals, including bio-identical hormones.

If your doctor is reluctant or uncomfortable dealing with natural hormones, I would recommend going directly to the compound pharmacy and having them recommend a physician who would be amenable to using natural hormones.

I remember the days when my patients would be yelled at by their gynecologists because they came to see me. These doctors would get angry because I took their patients off estrogen; they would literally throw their patients' natural hormone creams in the garbage. Needless to say, these doctors are now beginning to realize that they may have been mistaken.

PROGESTERONE

This is the number one hormone that has to be replaced. Please note: doctors will often state that if you do not have a uterus, you do not need progesterone. This is 100% wrong. The benefits of natural progesterone are repeated throughout this book. It is used as a transdermal cream that is absorbed through the skin fairly rapidly. Giving hormones by cream allows them to bypass the liver on the first go-around. When progesterone reaches the liver, it is converted into a different form of progesterone.

The problem with oral progesterone, as recommended in Suzanne Somers' book, *The Sexy Years*, is that it goes directly to the liver and gets converted. The same thing happens with the oral progesterone called Prometrium. This too is bio-identical, but converts to a different hormone.

Progesterone cream has to be applied to areas where the skin is thin because you want it going in to the blood stream, not fatty tissue. The best place is the wrist area and lower forearm (the inside, not the outside). Another site could be the upper chest (not breast). It should never be applied to the abdomen or thighs.

The prescription should read: Progesterone 100 mg/¼ tsp. Apply ¼ tsp BID. I recommend that it be used twice a day, every day, morning and evening.

Please note: Some women experience nipple tenderness when first starting progesterone. There are many progesterone receptor sites around the nipples. If this occurs, lower the dosage to 1/8 tsp, and later on go back up to ¼ tsp dose as the tenderness diminishes.

Some women experience menstrual bleeding after starting progesterone. Progesterone does not cause bleeding, but it does heal the uterus. The only hormone that causes bleeding is estrogen and, if estrogen levels are high enough, bleeding may occur. But this too will pass after one or two months.

THE TREATMENT OF ESTROGEN DOMINANCE

Prior to the menopause, all symptoms related to an overproduction of estrogen can be eliminated using natural progesterone. These symptoms include: menstrual cramps, breast tenderness, PMS, migraine headaches, mood swings, asthma, etc. The dosage here is the same as for menopause— 100mg/¼ teaspoon twice a day. For those patients who feel more comfortable mimicking how the body naturally produces hormones, you can omit the first seven to ten days after your cycle starts. This is necessary as well for those women wishing to get pregnant.

FERTILITY

One of the areas I believe that represents a tragic lack of hormonal knowledge is in the field of fertility. Please note the following:

1. The number one reason why women fail to get pregnant or have trouble getting pregnant is a low progesterone level

2. The number one reason why women have miscarriages is a low progesterone level

3. The only reason women experience nausea when they are pregnant is a low progesterone level (the nausea is actually caused by estrogen)

4. A frequent cause of premature birth is a low progesterone level

5. The only cause of post-partum depression, also known as the "baby blues," is a drop in progesterone levels

For those women interested in becoming proactive about their problems with fertility, conception and maintaining their pregnancies, natural progesterone is often the answer. For those who wish to avoid the expense and pain of in vitro fertilization, why not try natural progesterone?

The uterus requires progesterone for the fertilized egg to implant. It requires progesterone to sustain the pregnancy. Cramps, PMS, and breast tenderness with the monthly cycle—

all are classic symptoms indicative of low progesterone levels. Giving natural progesterone not only eliminates these symptoms, but heals the uterus and allows pregnancy to occur.

The dosage is 100mg/¼ tsp—twice a day, applied topically to the forearm/wrist. I would recommend using it daily for two months to get the uterus healed. At the onset of the third cycle, stop the progesterone for 10 days, and then restart it. If you become pregnant, you must increase the amount of progesterone as soon as you know that conception has occurred. This is best done with the use of a vaginal suppository, in the dose of 400 mg twice a day, which must be maintained for at least four months, if not longer, and ideally, throughout the whole pregnancy. Use it frequently enough to prevent nausea. Around the fourth or fifth month the placenta starts pouring out progesterone so you can discontinue it, but it may be wise to continue it.

The use of high dosages of progesterone after you're pregnant will provide three exceptional benefits: 1) no feelings of nausea, 2) prevention of miscarriage, and 3) an exceptionally intelligent, usually very happy baby. Progesterone is exceptionally important for brain function development. Certainly, premature infants might benefit from progesterone, since they are prematurely deprived of the normally high levels of progesterone put out by the placenta in the 2nd and 3rd trimesters.

REPLACEMENT OF POST/PERIMENOPAUSAL ESTROGEN

There are three different estrogen compounds produced by the body: estradiol, estrone and estriol, listed from the strongest to the weakest.

Please keep in mind that my approach to hormone

replacement for women is a very personal one. My mother died of breast cancer and had been on estrogen therapy, so perhaps I have a personal distaste for estrogen. My recommendations are based mostly on logic, somewhat on intuition and a lot on personal experience with thousands of patients.

I will try to list the different categories that women fall into and will explain my approach to each one.

PERIMENOPAUSAL/EARLY MENOPAUSE

This is a time when lab tests are helpful. My preferred approach is to try to eliminate any hot flashes or night sweats without using estrogen. Replacement of certain natural hormones at this time can often eliminate menopausal symptoms, especially replacing progesterone, testosterone or dehydroepiendosterone (DHEA).

A recommended hormone panel would include:

- Progesterone
- Estradiol
- DHEA-S
- Free testosterone

If a woman is still having periods, the ideal time to do a panel is about 7 days prior to the onset of her cycle. If symptoms are mild, I will start with progesterone cream, possibly testosterone cream and possibly DHEA.

If symptoms are severe, I will add BiEst Cream (combination of 20% estradiol and 80% estriol); 1.25 mg/¼ tsp. This can be applied to the skin once or twice a day. As soon as the symptoms abate, I recommend that the dosage be continuously decreased. The eventual aim is to stop the hormone if possible.

If women do not have a major problem with hot flashes,

but do have vaginal dryness, then I prescribe estriol cream; 2.5 mg/¼ tsp. along with a vaginal applicator. This is applied intra-vaginally on a daily basis until the dryness is gone, then it is used perhaps once every week or every other week, depending on dryness.

Again, please keep in mind that women never stop making estrogen. It is manufactured by fat cells, skin cells and the adrenal glands. There are women who feel better with the replacement of estrogen. However, the majority of women I have treated have not required it.

FOR THOSE WOMEN ON ESTROGEN

In spite of what most doctors think, the only clinical reason for replacing estrogen is to achieve levels of estrogen high enough to enable a woman to get pregnant. There are no benefits to the human body that I am aware of for high estrogen levels except to achieve conception.

By giving high levels of estrogen, especially for years, the pituitary has been tricked into thinking the woman is still trying to get pregnant. Stopping estrogen at this point often results in severe hot flashes, night sweats, etc. Very often, coming off Premarin is like detoxing off heroin.

In these cases it is often necessary to maintain estrogen in the form of BiEst Cream 1.25 mg/¼ tsp., used twice a day to start and gradually trying to wean off of it.

This, of course, is used in conjunction with the other missing hormones: progesterone, DHEA and testosterone.

Again, let me repeat, women never stop making estrogen—admittedly, not high enough levels to get them pregnant. However, if this is your goal, take the advice of Suzanne Somers' physician and take high levels of estrogen. Of course, since there are no eggs left, getting pregnant will be tough. It has been my observation that women who are thin are more likely to benefit and /or require estrogen since they have fewer fat cells to produce it. Women who are over-weight are generally loath to take it because in most cases, giving any type of estrogen prevents them from burning fat and losing weight.

THE 2ND MOST IMPORTANT HORMONE

After progesterone, the most necessary hormone to be replaced in women is testosterone. Just like estrogen, women continue to make testosterone, but at reduced levels. When evaluating testosterone levels, the free testosterone level (this is the biologically active form of testosterone) is usually around 1.6. This compares to a level of 6.4 during the teenage years.

The benefits of testosterone are manifold. This is the number one hormone needed by the bones and necessary for the prevention and treatment of osteoporosis. It is also the number one hormone for heart health. There are more testosterone receptor sites in heart muscle than anywhere else in the body. There are 250,000 deaths attributed to congestive heart failure (weakening of the heart muscle) every year. How many of these deaths might be avoided with the use of testosterone?

In addition, testosterone is probably the most important hormone for prevention of Alzheimer's disease. Also, you cannot build muscles without the use of testosterone. The more muscles one has, the more one is able to prevent fat from forming and skin from sagging.

A woman requires two hormones for a good libido (an interest in sex)—progesterone and testosterone. After starting these hormones, it may take about six weeks for the libido to kick in.

TESTOSTERONE AND URINARY INCONTINENCE

A very common problem in many women is the occurrence of urinary incontinence. Anytime they cough, sneeze, laugh in public, or run on the tennis court, urine dribbles out. This forces many women to resort to mini-pads. Discussions with their doctors lead to their receiving prescriptions for Detrol or Ditropan, drugs that focus on bladder function. At times they are referred to urologists for bladder surgery. Quite often, perhaps more often than not, the medication and the surgery do not help. The reason for this is that usually the incontinence they are experiencing is not a bladder problem. As women get older, the muscles around the urethra weaken and they cannot keep urine from leaking out of the bladder.

Using natural testosterone cream is almost 100% effective for this problem. The bio-identical testosterone cream is obtained from a compound pharmacy along with a vaginal applicator. The proper amount is inserted vaginally once a day in the morning. There are two sets of exercises that <u>must be done </u>to insure effectiveness. The first exercise is the Kegel exercise—this is the process of stopping and starting the stream while you are urinating. These are the exact muscles you are trying to build up. The second set of exercises is done during the day, primarily in the morning. The same muscles used for the Kegel maneuver need to be compressed for about ten seconds, 20 to 30 times per day. This can be done while you're driving, sitting and watching television, etc.

In about six to seven days, most women will experience 100% resolution of the incontinence—if they do <u>both sets </u>of exercises. Once the incontinence is gone, the testosterone cream can be applied to the inner forearm.

Dosages:

First month—2% cream or gel, 1/8 tsp (½ gm.), applied

intra vaginally (if necessary for incontinence) or 1/8 tsp to the forearm. Second month and thereafter—1% cream or gel, 1/8 tsp applied to the forearm on a daily basis.

The best way to gauge testosterone is by the libido. If you are experiencing a healthy libido, cut the dosage to two or three times per week. Too much testosterone can create side effects—acne, body hair growth, scalp hair loss, elevated cholesterol and aggressive behavior, etc. When dealing with hormones one must remember that these are powerful chemicals and they should be monitored carefully. However, used correctly, the benefits always outweigh the downside.

DHEA—THE ANTI-AGING HORMONE

Forty percent of DHEA (Dehydroepiendosterone) is made by the ovaries. Prior to and after the menopause, the ovaries quit manufacturing this hormone. It is considered the mother of steroid hormones, since it is the precursor to other hormones, most notably estrogen and testosterone. It is readily apparent that replacement of this hormone by itself can lead to a diminishment of hot flashes and night sweats and can help to restore libido. DHEA is known as an anti-aging hormone. There appears to be a direct correlation between levels of DHEA and longevity. People with the highest DHEA levels seem to live a long time. Perhaps this might be related to the fact that DHEA stimulates the production of growth hormone, sometimes referred to as the "fountain of youth" hormone.

The primary source of DHEA is the adrenal gland. People who have been exposed to high levels of stress during their life very often have low levels of DHEA.

DHEA influences the immune system and helps prevent cancer and arthritis. It's also beneficial to the cardiovascular system. It has the same effect as the "good" cholesterol (HDL) on the "bad" cholesterol (LDL), in that it prevents its oxidation, which can cause damage to the coronary arteries.

It is also known as a fat-burning hormone. The most likely reason for its weight loss promoting ability is that it lowers insulin levels, just like progesterone and testosterone.

It has the tendency to enhance one's feeling of well-being. However, as with any other hormone, the replacement should be correlated carefully with the need. Because this hormone can convert into other hormones, it is absolutely necessary to check blood levels of this hormone prior to starting its use and to monitor them during usage.

Since DHEA levels change with age, so-called normal levels are fairly low after the menopause. My preference is to replace DHEA to achieve levels consistent with those levels found in women about 40 years of age. This level is in the neighborhood of about 250 to 300. I start those women with a level that is very low, around 30 or less, with a dosage of 25 mg a day. In women with levels around 100, I start with 12 ½ mg a day. My recommendation is that DHEA should be obtained by prescription from a compound pharmacy. You will be assured of receiving a pharmaceutical dosage in a sustained-release form. Buying DHEA over the counter is a crap-shoot. Standards for regulating dosages are low or non-existent. Hormones are potent chemicals and one should be careful with the usage.

The most common side effect of DHEA is acne. This usually indicates that most of the DHEA is being converted into testosterone.

The remedy here, of course, is to cut back on dosage or frequency of administration.

Please note: When measuring DHEA levels, always check DHEA-S levels rather than DHEA.

CHAPTER 24

PERMANENT WEIGHT LOSS

From the beginning of my clinical career, my approach to medicine has been preventive. It always made a lot more sense to me to prevent disease rather than to treat it.

As an internist, I was continuously dealing with patients concerned about their weight. As I observed those coping with obesity, it became clear that this condition wreaked havoc on many levels. If my patients could manage their weight, the task of creating overall wellness would be eased greatly. In other words, I found that weight management fit easily into a preventive medicine category.

From the outset I was struck by these interesting statistics:

- 98 percent of people who lose weight gain it all back again within five years

- Obesity is the second leading preventable cause
  of death (smoking is number one)

What if there was a type of cancer that had a 98% relapse rate after it was treated? Patients would not be happy with that type of success rate for a cancer. They would demand an alternative approach.

But for the last 50 years, Americans have bought into the traditional, time-worn medical advice that "you have to diet, exercise, and watch your fat intake" in order to manage your weight. Sound familiar?

By now you should have an understanding of my point of view about weight management, including my conviction that embarking on a weight loss program entails more than determination and will power. Balancing one's hormones, eliminating certain drugs, and a fundamental knowledge of certain nutritional guidelines set the stage for a successful approach to weight loss and wellness.

In this final chapter I will provide you with a logical understanding of how to achieve permanent weight loss.

THE DISEASE CALLED OBESITY

I feel that a major cause of our current epidemic of obesity is that physicians have been reluctant to look at obesity as a disease rather than as an eating problem. Doctors have an absolutely clear understanding that conditions like hypertension and diabetes, etc., are real diseases that cannot be managed using will power. They have no reluctance about helping their patients manage these conditions, even if it means treating them over their entire life span.

But obesity, they feel, can be treated with unsophisticated advice, with no efforts to address the underlying cause. If it's not a disease, why look for a cause? This is like trying to treat a cancer without treating the cause of the cancer.

I prefer a more scientific method. Let's look at the traditional approaches to weight management to get an understanding of why they don't work.

WHY CUTTING CALORIES DOESN'T WORK

The problem with calorie restriction (dieting) as a weight loss strategy is that it triggers the body's survival mechanisms. When we limit our meal plans to 1,200 or 1,500 calories per day, the body gets alarmed. Is starvation in the offing? Best to start storing and locking away fat in earnest.

The body is a complex, multi-layered operating system. It has a whole arsenal of techniques for maintaining homeostasis and for ensuring survival. This is something that dieters forget. They become fixated on counting calories, assuming that a body deprived of energy will burn its own fat to survive. But they are wrong. A body deprived of energy will go after its own muscle tissue before it will burn fat. And in the meantime, it will marshal its very powerful hormone system to alter the way it metabolizes food for energy.

People who lose weight on a diet are fooling themselves. They get on the scale and see that they weigh less, but they shouldn't be celebrating. They've just burned up muscle tissue—the only kind of tissue that burns fat. Now they have a body that's less efficient at burning fat. When they "finish" their diet (i.e. stop restricting calories) they will have less of the tissue needed to maintain homeostasis at a low weight.

As most people know, it's standard for people who diet to not only gain back all the weight they've lost, but to put on an extra two or three pounds. Lost muscle tissue—and the body's newly improved fat-storing mechanism—is what causes them to stabilize at a higher weight.

WHAT ABOUT EXERCISE?

Many people reason that if restricting calories is unrealistic, then the solution is to exercise more. Exercise, after all, burns calories.

Or does it?

Exercise offers tremendous benefits to those who incorporate it into their lifestyle. It improves cardiovascular health, it makes people feel better, it's great for bones and muscles, it lowers insulin levels, and so on. However, as the sole approach to weight loss it's not what it's cracked up to be.

To lose one pound of fat by exercising, you must burn 3,500 calories. This is equivalent to going out and running 35 miles. The alternative would be walking on a treadmill at 4 miles per hour for 7 1/2 hours.

In my practice I have come upon patients who were living on 800 calories a day and exercising four hours a day and they couldn't lose an ounce. Talk about frustrated! These people obviously were in a severe starvation mode, and the body will not burn fat when it's starving.

EATING LESS FAT

Another timeworn piece of advice was to tell patients to cut out fat from their diets. Interestingly, fat is the only food substance that does not stimulate insulin. And insulin, as most of you know, is the number one hormone that creates fat, especially around the middle.

Ever since this country got into a nonfat, fat-free thinking mode, we have had an epidemic of obesity. Foods like popcorn and pretzels, which are nonfat and low in calories, create more insulin than candy does. (However, the message here is not to eat candy.)

As reported in the Framingham Heart Study, which is the largest on-going heart study in the world, they found that those men who ate the most saturated fat (butter, meat, eggs, etc.) had the least weight problems. Additionally, they had the lowest cholesterol levels and the least coronary artery disease. Fat is not the enemy.

Additionally, if fat is the preferred fuel for survival, will the body burn it if a person restricts their fat intake? Very importantly, one must understand that foods that are nonfat are usually high in carbohydrates (sugar) which causes insulin levels to increase. Fat is the only food substance that does not stimulate insulin.

NOW WHAT? THE LOGICAL APPROACH

So we've eliminated dieting, we've eliminated exercise and we've eliminated eating less fat. Now what are we going to do?

Well, it all comes down to metabolism. The trick is to convert your body from a sugar-burning metabolism to a fat-burning metabolism. The way to do this is to take away sugar. The body gets sugar from carbohydrates. All carbohydrates break down into sugar. You must eliminate those particular carbohydrates that create the most sugar and/or stimulate the most insulin production.

It takes three days from the time you stop taking in sugar and certain other carbohydrates for your body to begin burning fat. It takes that long to get the sugar, or glycogen, out of the muscle tissue. Once you get rid of glycogen, the usual source of energy, the muscles have no choice: they have to start burning fat. After that point, everything you do burns fat. Cleaning the house, walking out to the car, walking your dog, everything you do burns fat. Even while you are sleeping, you are burning fat.

You're still up against that 3,500 calories that it takes to lose a pound of fat, but now you are burning fat constantly. For most people, depending upon how much they weigh and how active they are, this allows them to burn anywhere from 7,000 to 10,000 calories per week So the expected fat loss using this type of approach would be anywhere from two to three pounds per week, or eight to twelve pounds per month.

SAYING GOODBYE TO INSULIN

Obviously this type of approach is not for everybody. However, there are certain types of people who have no other choice except to follow this plan.

These are the people who:

- Are not big eaters. They can't shave 3,500 calories from their meal plans in order to lose one pound of fat.

- Over-produce insulin

- Have Syndrome X

- Have low progesterone levels

- Eat too much sugar

For most people, insulin is the enemy. Insulin creates *fat* by taking any sugar the muscles have no need for and placing it into fat cells, where the sugar is immediately converted into fat. Then insulin sits there preventing release of fat from the fat cells—it is a fat-storing hormone.

The bottom line for most people is that to get rid of fat you have to get rid of insulin. If you want to get rid of insulin, you have to take away sugar. Sugar stimulates insulin production.

SIMILAR APPROACHES

This is the basic premise behind many weight loss approaches: Atkins, The South Beach Diet, Sugar Busters, The Zone, Protein Power, the Carbohydrate Addict's Diet, the Mayo Clinic Diet, the Grapefruit Diet, Stillman…it goes on and on.

What used to be a low-fat world is rapidly converting into a low-carb world. Many restaurants offer low-carb menus, and fast food places have also jumped on the band wagon.

This concept of eating low carb is not new. It has actually been around for about 156 years. There were several successful low carb programs in the 1800's, which eventually died out. The idea was resurrected in the 1970's by Stillman and Atkins. Now there are low carb gurus everywhere. The approach is not for everyone, but it definitely is for people who over-produce insulin. This probably includes about 90% of people who are over-weight.

One must be aware that each particular diet plan is not for everybody—there is no "one-size-fits-all" approach. For example, one diet plan allows a "reward meal" at supper (eat as many carbohydrates as you want within the space of an hour). People with hyperinsulinemia—which is perhaps the majority of people with weight problems—will not be successful on this meal plan. I had a patient for whom a half cup of split pea soup would prevent her from burning fat for seven days. For some people, one piece of bread, one carrot stick, or one yam will prevent fat-burning for three days.

Other low-carbohydrate plans give people the impression they can eat as much protein as they want. But this is misleading. The body cannot store protein. Any excess protein the body can't use or eliminate is converted into sugar for fat storage. In this situation, you can be burning fat (i.e., be in ketosis) and be storing fat at the same rate and you will not be losing weight.

ADDITIONAL THOUGHTS ON WEIGHT LOSS

In order for the body to burn fat, you have to feed it and water it. The first requirement means that you cannot skip any meals. The body requires fuel 24 hours a day: your heart is beating, you're breathing, and there are thousands of chemical reactions occurring all of the time. When you skip breakfast, you are going without fuel for 15 hours. The body will now automatically store fat for the next 24 hours. So even if you are not hungry, you still have to eat.

The other requirement is water. Fifty percent of your body is water. You cannot burn fat without water. Water is important. Keep an eye on the color of your urine. If it's yellow, you're dehydrated. Drink more water. Try to get your urine as clear as possible.

Alcohol does not enhance weight loss. The body likes alcohol as a fuel. It's an easy fuel to burn and it burns at seven calories per gram, almost as much as fat. Given the choice, the body will always burn alcohol before fat. The bottom line: if you want your body to burn fat, don't give it alcohol.

There is an old wives' tale that says if you want to lose weight, you have to give up coffee. In actuality, caffeine may stimulate insulin production, but not in everybody. People with Syndrome X (high insulin, high triglycerides, and low

HDL cholesterol) traditionally have the worst problem with caffeine in terms of insulin.

There are strips called Ketostix that are available in any drugstore. You can use them to find out whether you are burning fat. The end-stage of fat metabolism produces ketone bodies that are partially eliminated through the kidneys. If you have ketone bodies in your urine, these Ketostix will change color indicating you are burning fat. Everyone's metabolism is different, so using Ketostix will help you to find out what you can get away with in your meal plan.

CORTISOL AND WEIGHT

There has been a lot of attention in the last year or two to the relationship of cortisol to fat. Listening to the advertisements on the radio and television, one could almost surmise that this is the only cause of weight problems. Let me try to put it in perspective so you will have a better understanding. People who are trying to lose weight must realize that they are dealing with a body whose main function in life is survival. In accordance with this, the body has become extremely efficient over the years at creating and storing fat, which it considers the most important fuel for survival.

To aid in survival, the body also has the adrenal glands, which produce hormones at times of extreme stress to help the body either fight a predator or escape. This system worked pretty well in the cave man days. After seeing a sabre-tooth tiger, the adrenal glands would produce cortisol, which would raise sugar levels to give the muscles energy for fight or flight, and they would release adrenalin to give additional energy or stimulate fat cells to release fat for even more energy. However, this system was set up for a stress reaction lasting about 10 minutes.

In this day and age, people get subjected to stress continuously—at work, driving, meeting schedules, etc. In these situations, the adrenal glands may be continuously putting out cortisol, which is continuously raising sugar levels, which is continuously raising insulin levels, which is continuously creating fat.

Whether or not cortisol is a major source of weight problems in people, I am not convinced. Suffice to say, however, that high cortisol levels do not promote weight loss.

Stress is never good for the body. The more in balance you are with your hormones, and your environment, the healthier you will be. Look for areas in your life giving negative energy, and eliminate them. Eliminate time constraints, if you can. Say "no" to road rage.

One last thing: exercise is a great way to reduce excess adrenal hormones and reduce stress, and maybe help with weight loss.

THE MAINTENANCE PHASE

In my practice, when patients reach goal weight they enter the second phase of the program, which is geared toward preventing fat from returning to the body. As long as a person limits the amount of carbohydrates to the amount of sugar required by muscle tissue, excess carbohydrates will not be stored as fat. In this regard, the amount of exercise a person is involved with is the main determinant of weight maintenance. The body's priority is to replace any sugar that the muscles have burned, back to the muscles—it's a survival thing. The more sugar (glycogen) the muscles have burned, the more of the carbohydrates you eat will go into muscle rather than being stored as fat.

If people do not want to exercise, they have to be more aware of their carbohydrate intake. People who produce excess insulin because of Syndrome X may require medication (e.g., metformin, also known as Glucophage) or supplements (e.g., chromium, alpha lipoic acid, etc.) to lower their insulin levels.

However, getting one's hormones back into balance and eliminating fat-creating medications is perhaps the key to successful weight maintenance. Here the most important hormones are progesterone and thyroid.

THE MISSING FACTORS

As stated earlier, statistically 98% of people gain weight back after losing it, regardless of the approach they have used. This includes Weight Watchers, Jenny Craig, Lindora, Atkin's and gastric bypass. As soon as people get off any program they have followed, the weight comes back on. The reason for this is that the underlying mechanism that created the fat in the first place is still there, whether it be an over-production of insulin, an under active thyroid, too much estrogen or other lipogenic (fat-creating) drugs, etc.

If these factors are not addressed, your body will always be creating too much fat. Throughout this book I have introduced you to a number of my patients who had a lifetime of frustration until these factors were taken into consideration.

A SIMPLE PHILOSOPHY

My method for successful, permanent weight loss is simple. It's based on principles that have been around for a long time and have worked for many people. But it will not work unless the body's hormones are in balance.

Since hormone levels decrease as we age, the older you are, the likelier it is that you may need to have your hormones adjusted. For reasons discussed throughout this book, finding a doctor who can balance your hormones successfully, using the natural hormones that involve the fewest side effects, isn't easy. I hope I've provided enough information, hints and examples in this book to help you in your quest to receive proper treatment with natural hormones. And perhaps now you have a better understanding of how your body operates, so you may be in control of your health and wellness.

FINAL THOUGHT

A philosopher once said that all new ideas must go through three phases. First, they are ridiculed. Next, they are viciously attacked. Finally, way down the line, they are accepted as self-evident truths. At this point, doctors will say, "Yes, we've known this all along."

FOR MORE INFORMATION CONTACT:

Michael E. Platt, M.D.
73-345 Highway 111, Suite 203
Palm Desert, CA 92260

- Phone 760.836.3232 Toll Free 877-Dr-Platt
- Fax 760.836.3234
- Email: questions@drplatt.com
- Website: www.drplatt.com

GO TO DR. PLATT'S WEBSITE FOR:

- Your Free Hormone Evaluation Online
- Lifestyle Evaluation
- Weight Loss Information

GO TO DR. PLATT'S WEBSITE TO SEE

DR. PLATT'S VIDEO

www.drplatt.com

If you would like to find a Compounding Pharmacy near your home, you may call: 877-340-5922.

INDEX